Functional Fitness

The Personal Trainer's Guide

Lamar Lowery

FUNCTIONAL FITNESS

THE PERSONAL TRAINER'S GUIDE

Meyer & Meyer Sport

British Library Cataloguing in Publication Data
A catalogue record for this book is available from the British Library

Original title: Functional Fitness – That's It! Lamars beste Workouts und Trainingspläne
Translation: AAA Translations, St. Louis, Missouri

Functional Fitness. The Personal Trainer's Guide
Maidenhead: Meyer & Meyer Sport (UK) Ltd., 2016
ISBN 978-1-78255-094-5

© 2016 by Meyer & Meyer Sport (UK) Ltd.
Aachen, Auckland, Beirut, Cairo, Cape Town, Dubai, Hägendorf, Hong Kong,
Indianapolis, Manila, New Delhi, Singapore, Sydney, Tehran, Vienna

 Member of the World Sport Publishers' Association (WSPA)

Manufacturing: Print Consult GmbH, München
E-Mail: info@m-m-sports.com
www.m-m-sports.com

TABLE OF CONTENTS

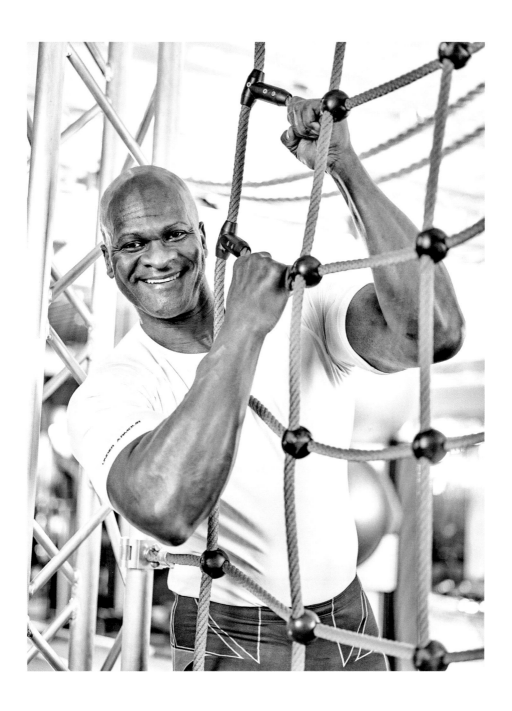

CHAPTER 1

INTRODUCTION
–
WHO IS LAMAR LOWERY?

INTRODUCTION – WHO IS LAMAR LOWERY?

When you see me, Lamar Lowery, you will inevitably think of an action figure that has come to life. As a six-foot, five-inch American model athlete with dual German-American citizenship, I am a constant commuter between the old and the new world. My job: personal trainer.

For 38 years, I, Lamar Lowery, born in Manhattan, NY in 1966, have been training athletes, executives, and many other groups of people, with innovative training methods built around functional fitness. I was convinced from the start that a structured approach—by the way, a rather German mindset—determination, and regular continued education, or rather, information, in the areas of training, tactics, and research can produce great results in the health and wellness industry. I have always considered this tenet in my own training.

CAREER

- 1984 graduated from high school
- Benedict College 1984-1988/BA Sports Science
- Columbia Junior College/Midlands
- Technical College/Athletic scholarships

❯ 1986-1989 South Carolina Department of Lexington County Mental Health Hospital, Columbia, South Carolina
❯ Mental health specialist as a male nursing assistant
❯ 1989-1994 service in the U.S. Army
❯ Army master of physical fitness
❯ Instructor and master instructor
❯ Fitness Institute International, Inc./exercise science foundations course
❯ Fitness testing specialist course
❯ Functional training specialist course
❯ Nutrition education and weight management specialist course
❯ Special populations/post-rehab specialist course
❯ Strength and conditioning specialist course
❯ CPTS
❯ Fascia training level 1
❯ Fascia training level 2

TRAINER ACTIVITY
1995-2000 World Sport West End, Wetzlar, Germany
          Maritim Hotel, Frankfurt, Germany
          Hilton Hotel, Frankfurt, Germany

PERSONAL TRAINER
2000-2003 part-time coaching
2003-2005 Personal Training Company, Palm Beach, Florida

HARMONY TRAINING WITH LAMAR
2005-2007 MS in Sales Representative Consulting & Training GmbH, Wetzlar, Germany

PERSONAL TRAINER
2007 founding of the Lamar Functional Training Academy

I have always dreamt of having my own training facility. For 15 years, I have been a successful personal trainer in Germany, have been working with the leaders of large companies as well as many celebrities, and have been a contributor to trade journals. Eight years ago, I founded the Lamar Functional Training Academy. "My" functional training is comprised of individual exercises that are specifically geared to the client's respective activities. My clients include the very busy Frankfurt executive as well as the successful businesswoman from Gießen or the retiree who wants to improve his golf handicap.

To me, as a health professional, a good education, a well-trained eye, and lots of experience are the most important qualifications for the success of clients and trainers. Thanks to these foundations I am also able to help those recovering after an operation or injury to eliminate pain. Many people suffering from back pain feel fit, healthy, and resilient again after a specific workout with me. I live by my conviction: Targeted functional training is the best training for everyday life.

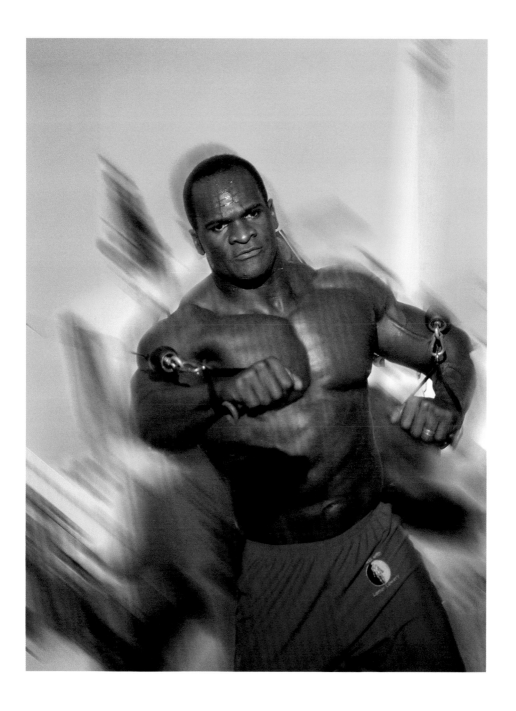

CHAPTER 2

FUNCTIONAL TRAINING

FUNCTIONAL TRAINING

Functional training is not new; rather we have encountered it for several years, and it is probably one of the currently most overused terms in the fitness industry. An Internet search of functional training will produce 23,600,000 hits.

In the fitness industry there is the phenomenon of the market pendulum trending heavily in a certain direction on the spectrum of offerings. Currently it is the area of functional training. There was a time when many trainers used what I like to call the "Cirque de Soleil" training method. The philosophy behind this method excoriated any training exercise less complex than a one-armed shoulder press with a dumbbell while standing on one leg on a BOSU balance trainer as not functional and not suitable for everyday life. The problem with this philosophy is twofold. For one, the likelihood of executing a one-armed shoulder press with a weight while standing on one leg on an unstable surface is relatively low in everyday life, and, secondly, the more instability we add to an exercise, the smaller the load we can tolerate.

This type of training allows us to overload the central nervous system but hardly allows us to overload the musculature to create the necessary training stimulus—an example of a concept that could have some value but was overused. The reaction to this extreme philosophy was a big swing of the pendulum in the opposite direction. Suddenly the use of stability balls and balance boards in training was viewed in a negative light, and some trainers and therapists completely banished useful training aids from their sphere of activity.

While many people tend to believe that there is only one superior form of training and everything else that doesn't fit this philosophy is of no value, I believe that there are and should be many different effective forms of training. Anything that helps us reach our goals should be used. When I talk about functional fitness, I talk about the ability to improve daily functionality through movement patterns that we humans use every day—simple, effective workouts without a safety net and false bottom.

The one-sided activities in our jobs and recreation often result in a general lack of movement along with poor posture, decreased fitness, and, thereby, lower quality of life. The current trend is "back to the roots," away from extreme sports and exaggerated weight loss, back to balanced exercise where the focus is on increased well-being and disease prevention.

My functional training draws on tried and tested training principles and combines them in an efficient manner. It adopts the body's natural tasks, its movements and functions, and practices movement patterns from everyday life to balance body, spirit, and soul and to preserve that balance long-term.

The goal of functional training is to "wake up" the body and give it mobility for life. This is done through

❱ targeted movement of ideally all of the body's muscles and joints,
❱ targeted movement and activation of the spine,
❱ activation of the neurological system,
❱ activation of the nervous system, and
❱ activation of the muscular system.

The exercises in my functional training program make people stronger, more powerful, and draw from many training philosophies. My long-time international experience in fitness training and ongoing exchange with personal trainers in the US make my concept unique. This book provides an insight into my world of functional fitness training.

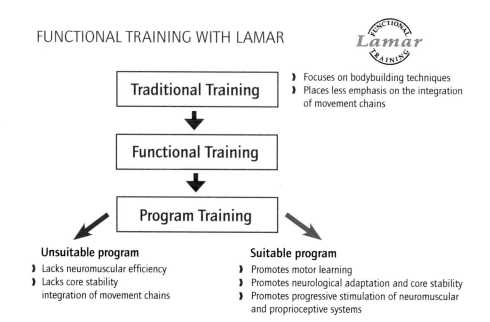

Fig. 1: Functional training with Lamar

2.1   DEFINITION

Functional training is a revolutionary training method from the US with ancient roots. Functional training can be labeled as the latest hype or as the catchphrase of the sports scene. At the same time, the content of this form of training is still hotly debated. The best way to define this form of training is to take a closer look at the original meaning of the individual words.

Function can be defined as **carrying out an action** for which a person is specifically equipped or intended for. Meaning, a function has a specific purpose.

Training, on the other hand, denotes a complex process that induces an altered development by processing stimuli. In summary, you could say that functional training develops or practices movements the body was built for with the goal of achieving an altered, ideally improved, sense of well-being, meaning purposeful training. But purposeful is relative because it is always subject to the individual situation. Thus, we can train a mason so he is able to execute his activities of heavy lifting, bending, stretching, and diagonal reaching particularly effectively, while the older woman needs the necessary leg strength and coordination to walk up the stairs to her third-floor apartment, and the elite soccer player needs, next to speed, strength and endurance, particularly good reaction ability, and ball coordination. All of these factors cannot be viewed as separate.

The human body is an extremely complex work of art. The constant interplay between different body systems and their individual parts enables the functions that define our lives. With its present-day "construction," adapted to its respective environment, the human body is the product of a long evolutionary process.

We must, therefore, also allow an individual scope for functional training—a scope that personal trainers such as I use for the benefit of the client and to achieve the best-possible results.

In summary, functional training has the following characteristics:
- everyday and sport specific
- individual, yet still specific
- versatile and varied
- progressive

In doing so, it follows five global principles:
1. Integrate, not isolate. Training complex movement sequences, meaning not just isolating individual muscles, but rather entire muscle chains the way they are also used in everyday life.
2. Multidimensional bandwidth. Training movement patterns from daily life (everyday life, job, sports) that require the use of multiple joints on different planes.
3. Quality over quantity.
4. Use the body's own stabilizers, especially core stability instead of external stabilizers, such as chairs or benches.
5. Address correctable compensations and dysfunctions.

Body awareness and coordination are important parts of training within all of these principles. There is also emphasis on muscle and joint mobility, areas that unfortunately still don't receive enough attention in some forms of training but that are very important for good quality of life and injury prevention in sports.

2.2 THE PHILOSOPHY BEHIND COMPLETE TRAINING – FUNDAMENTALS OF FUNCTIONAL FITNESS

We refer to the three main systems that essentially provide the functions of the human body in our daily lives: the central nervous system, the nervous system, and the muscle system. Another system, the skeletal system, should also be taken into account.

These systems form a kind of symbiosis. A comparison from the realm of technology would be the car in which one important part cannot function without another. For instance, the engine cannot work without the fuel supply and ignition system, which in turn cannot work without electricity, and the cooling system is also crucial. Then there is the transmission, the chassis, wheels, and tires. But the body and windows as well as the entire interior make no sense without the previously mentioned systems and are what makes a car a car with all of the functions we humans expect. If we removed all of the technology and its interconnectedness we would be left with the car's "nude body," the shell. We must, therefore, understand how important it is that each individual system functions, because each system becomes the problem of the whole if it does not function properly.

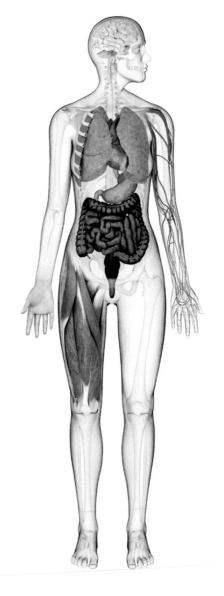

Fig. 2: The central nervous system, the nervous system, and the musculature as central systems of the human body

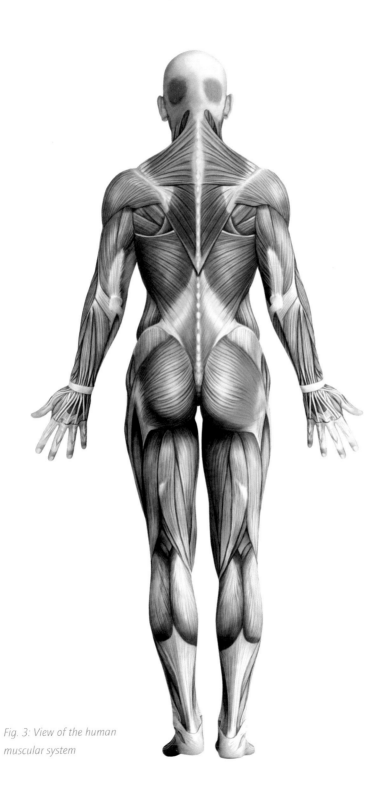

*Fig. 3: View of the human
muscular system*

To keep this interplay intact, the individual organs in the human body must be connected directly or indirectly, much like the wires and parts of a car. The skeleton that lends the body support and shape makes such connections possible. Nearly all organs are in contact with each other and, at the same time, are protected through a framework of cartilage and bone, which is also the comprehensive network of the fascia. Vital substances such as red blood cells for oxygen transport and mineral salts are provided courtesy of our bones. Moreover, lots of receptors in the fascia provide an extensive exchange of information.

2.2.1   MUSCULATURE

A more or less expansive chapter on anatomy, the individual muscle systems, and their functions could follow here. But since the focus of this book is training, I will at this time refer to existing literature dedicated strictly to that topic and will only briefly address those areas important to me and relevant to practical training.

The skeleton of an adult human is comprised of approximately 206 individual bones that are connected by real or artificial joints. Our body possesses about 650 muscles without which we would not be able to move.

It is unlikely that such a large number of muscles within the "intelligent" human system developed solely for inactivity and rest. On the contrary, the human system is genetically constructed for movement and continuous loading. Our musculature weighs more than our bone frame (i.e., skeleton). While muscle makes up about 40% of our body weight, the skeleton is only 14%. The interplay of muscular, skeletal, and nervous systems makes human motion possible.

Each of our movements or postures requires activity of certain muscles. Muscle movements can only take place in conjunction with the nervous system and the brain. Our sensory organs allow us to perceive stimuli and sensations that are transmitted to the brain through the nervous system. It reacts with the appropriate "orders" that are then transmitted to the muscles through the nervous system. Each of these muscles is a separate organ consisting of skeletal muscle tissue, blood vessels, tendons, and nerves. Muscle tissue can also be found in the heart, in the digestive organs, and in the blood vessels. In these organs, muscles are responsible for the transport of substances throughout the body. They are constantly active. They cannot be controlled deliberately. The respiratory muscles are one example. We cannot deliberately release them from their activity. We must, therefore, note that there are three types of muscle tissue:

- ❯ Visceral or involuntary (smooth) muscles
- ❯ Skeletal or voluntary (striated) muscles
- ❯ Heart muscle (special, striated muscle)

VISCERAL MUSCULATURE

Visceral musculature can be found in the organs—for instance, in the abdomen, in the colon, and in the blood vessels. It is the weakest muscle tissue, and it makes sure that organs contract for the transport of substances. Since visceral musculature cannot be controlled deliberately, it is also referred to as involuntary musculature. Due to its smooth, even appearance in microscopic images, it is also called smooth musculature. By contrast, heart and skeletal muscle is striped horizontally.

HEART MUSCLE

The heart muscle makes sure that blood is pumped throughout the body. It cannot be controlled deliberately and is, therefore, an involuntary muscle. The heart muscle activates itself and, thereby, contracts. But the contraction frequency is regulated by hormones and signals from the brain. The natural heart pacemaker consists of heart muscle tissue that activates other heart muscle cells, prompting them to contract. Due to this self-activation, the heart muscle's function is considered as autorhythmic, or its regulation as intrinsic.

The cells of the heart muscle are striped; when looking at them under a microscope they appear to have light and dark bands. These light and dark bands are created by the arrangement of protein fibers in the cells. The horizontal stripes indicate that the muscle cell is very strong contrary to the visceral musculature.

SKELETAL MUSCULATURE

Skeletal muscles are the only voluntary muscles in the human body and are controlled deliberately. Every physical activity an individual consciously performs (e.g., talking, walking, or writing) requires skeletal muscle. A skeletal muscle contracts to bring parts of the body closer to the bone to which it is attached. Most skeletal muscles are attached to two bones across a joint so the muscle is able to move parts of these bones closer together. Skeletal muscle cells form by many smaller precursor cells bundling together into long, straight, polynuclear fibers.

Like the heart muscle, skeletal muscles are striped horizontally, and skeletal muscle fibers are very strong. The name skeletal muscle stems from the fact that these muscles connect to the skeleton in at least one place.

RELEVANCE TO TRAINING – WHAT IS IMPORTANT?

When taking a closer look at the anatomical muscular system, it quickly becomes apparent that most muscles run diagonally or horizontally. The majority of trunk muscles (between the ischial tuberosity and the upper part of the sternum), more specifically 87.5%, run diagonally or horizontally. Their main function is movement. The following table shows the body is designed for rotational movement. Most trunk muscles are divided into vertical (no diagonal or rotational movement) and non-vertical (diagonal, horizontal, and rotational movement) muscle groups. Sometimes we differentiate between and refer to large and small muscles and the degree to which they participate in a rotation or support a rotation. Some leg muscles were included because they are connected to the pelvic floor and help to turn the body when it is on the ground.

When looking at the following chart, you can see that the body's main function is rotation. Yet standard training concepts give little or no consideration to rotation.

Table 1: Function and location of trunk muscles

MUSCLES	NON-VERTICAL	VERTICAL
DORSAL (back)		
Trapezius muscle (m. trapezius)	X	
Rhomboid muscle (m. rhomboideus major/minor)	X	
Latissimus dorsi (m. latissiumus dorsi)	X	
Erector spinae (m. erector spinae)		X
Quadratus lumborum (m. quadratus lumborum)	X	
Gluteus maximus (m. gluteus maximus)	X	
Gluteus medius (m. gluteus medius)	X	
Gluteus minimus (m. gluteus minimus)	X	
Tensor fasciae latae (m. tensor fasciae latae)		X
Hip rotator muscles	X (6x)	
VENTRAL (abdomen)		
Pectoralis major (m. pectoralis major)	X	
Pectoralis minor (m. pectoralis minor)	X	
Serratus anterior (m. serratus anterior)	X	
External oblique muscle (m. obliquus externus abdominis)	X	
Internal oblique muscle (m. obliquus internus abdominis)	X	
Rectus abdominis (m. rectus abdominis)		X

MUSCLES	NON-VERTICAL	VERTICAL
Transverse abdominal muscle (m. transversus abdominis)	X	
Psoas (m. psoas)	X	
Iliacus muscle (m. iliacus)	X	
Sartorius muscle (m. sartorius)	X	
Rectus femoris muscle (m. rectus femoris)		X
Abductors	X (4x)	
Pectineus muscle (m. pectineus)	X	
Gracilis muscle (m. gracilis)	X	
TOTAL	28 pairs = 56	4 pairs = 8

% rotator muscles = 87,5 %

The spiral is a universal element of our locomotor system. Our body is built based on the same functional principles. Therefore, nearly all training should include rotation as an important function.

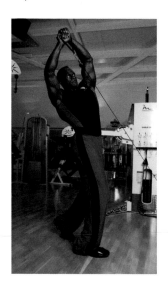

COMPLEXITY IN TRAINING

1. Posture
2. Coordination
3. Balance
4. Biomechanical axis
5. Speed
6. Strength components
7. Flexibility
8. Endurance

2.2.2 SKELETAL SYSTEM

Even though skeletons sometimes symbolize death and sinister, scary things, the skeleton is still one of the systems that lend the body life. Contrary to other living organs, bones are solid and strong, but they have their own blood and lymph vessels as well as nerves.

Bones consist of two different types of tissue:

❱ Compact bone tissue: This sturdy, compact tissue forms the outer layer of most bones and the sheath of long bones, such as in the arms and legs. Nerves and blood vessels can be found in this tissue.

❱ Sponge-like bone tissue: This tissue consists of smaller trabeculae with red bone marrow located in between. It is found at the ends of long bones (e.g., the head of the femur) and inside other bones.

A fully-grown human body has 206 bones of which nearly 50% are located in the hands and feet. Joints or interstices connect the bones to each other and lend our bodies stability and protection for all internal organs. We differentiate between fibrous, or osseous, joints that move very little or not at all and true joints with different ranges of motion, depending on the type of joint.

Many joints are able to move on all three planes simultaneously (see chapter 3.2). For instance, a joint can be flexed, pulled toward the body, and internally rotated, all at the same time. Even the small joints in the ankle complex can perform movements that we may not even be aware of. The following chart will help us to better understand functional movements.

SAGITTAL PLANE/VERTICAL – BACK TO FRONT MOTION

Table 2: Joint planes of motion

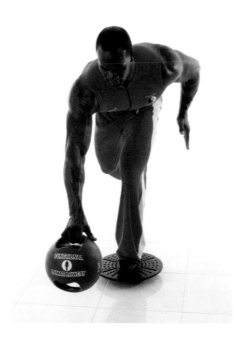

JOINT	MOTION
Hip	Flexion/extension
Knee	Flexion/extension
Ankle	Dorsal flexion/plantar flexion
Lower ankle joint	Dorsal flexion/plantar flexion
Midtarsal joint	Dorsal flexion/plantar flexion

FRONTAL PLANE – LEFT TO RIGHT MOTION

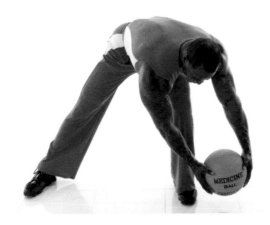

JOINT	MOTION
Hip	Abduction/adduction
Knee	Abduction/adduction
Ankle	–
Lower ankle (subtalar joint)	Inversion/eversion
Midtarsal joint	Inversion/eversion

TRANSVERSE PLANE – ROTATIONAL MOTION

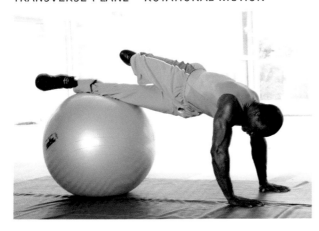

JOINT	MOTION
Hip	External/internal rotation
Knee	–
Ankle	–
Lower ankle (subtalar joint)	–
Midtarsal joint	–

PRONATION

JOINT	SAGITTAL	FRONTAL	TRANSVERSE
Hip	Flexion	Adduction	Internal rotation
Knee	Flexion	Abduction	Internal rotation
Ankle	Dorsal-/ Plantar flexion	–	Adduction/ abduction
Lower ankle	–	Eversion	Adduction
Midtarsal joint	Dorsal flexion	Inversion	Abduction

SUPINATION

GELENK	SAGITTAL	FRONTAL	TRANSVERSAL
Hip	Extension	Abduction	External rotation
Knee	Extension	Adduction	External rotation
Ankle	Dorsal-/ Plantar flexion	–	Adduction/ abduction
Lower ankle	–	–	Adduction
Midtarsal joint	Plantar flexion	–	Adduction

RELEVANCE TO TRAINING – WHAT IS IMPORTANT?

The joints are the human body's weak spot for anatomical reasons. Stability, mobility, and muscular control of joints should, therefore, be taken into account during training. The joint-encompassing muscles form a kind of "protective wall" that, with good neuromuscular control, can minimize or even prevent injuries.

2.2.3 CENTRAL NERVOUS SYSTEM

The central nervous system consists of the brain, spinal cord, and a complex neuronal network. This system is responsible for transmitting, receiving, and interpreting information from all parts of the body. The nervous system monitors and coordinates the function of internal organs and reacts to changes in the environment. It can be divided into two parts: the central nervous system and the peripheral nervous system.

The central nervous system (CNS) is the nervous system's processing center. It receives information from the peripheral nervous system and transmits information to the peripheral nervous system. The two main organs of the CNS are the brain and spinal cord. The brain processes and interprets sensory information transmitted by the spinal cord.

2.2.4 NERVOUS SYSTEM

The nervous system is a complex network of nerves and cells that transport messages to the brain and spinal cord and from the brain and spinal cord to other parts of the body.

The nervous system consists of the central and the peripheral nervous systems. The central nervous system consists of the brain and spinal cord, and the peripheral nervous system consists of the somatic and the vegetative nervous systems.

Neuromuscular control has a major impact on movement quality.

RELEVANCE TO TRAINING – WHAT IS IMPORTANT?

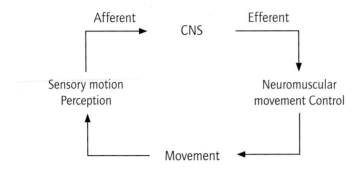

Fig. 4: Simplified illustration of the sensorimotor regulatory circuit as per Bruhn and Gollhofer (2001, p 66)

An interruption can result in the incorrect or uneconomical execution of movements. In the long term, these can be performance limiting or even lead to injuries. With sensorimotor training (see chapter 3.7), this can often be prevented.

2.3   WHAT CAN FUNCTIONAL TRAINING ACCOMPLISH?

Now we have heard much about functional training, but is this form of training just another "path to fitness" we must negotiate, or is it worth making a long-term commitment to our training and making it a part of our training practice? After 14 years of working as a trainer, I am convinced that incorporating functional training into our current training practice is one of the most important steps toward basic fitness and health. Anyone who thinks he can be successful without factoring in health is wrong. Physical training does not only affect the muscles but also well-being and performance capacity. Endurance, properly dosed strength, and flexibility are the cornerstones of physical performance. Traditional weightlifting usually only focuses on one muscle per exercise, whereas a functional exercise can work multiple body regions and, thereby, muscle chains.

In my opinion, the most relevant positive effects of personalized functional training are

> increased (inner) strength,
> endurance,
> improved, optimized basic stability along with flexibility (mobility),
> increased quality of life and balance, and
> improved body awareness.

These improvements result in increased performance capacity and decreased susceptibility to stress—important building blocks that all of us would like to list on the asset side of life.

Functional training makes muscles, fascia, and joints healthier and more stable, and just like we brush our teeth every day, we should do the same for our bodies and "remove the rust" through functional training.

Functional training works the muscles on different planes and, thus, from different angles. This targets stabilizing as well as fixator muscles. Gym equipment is preset and only allows the body to move within the preset angles and planes. In addition, the upper and lower body are often trained separately, which does not take into account the trunk as a stabilizing waypoint. Multiplane exercises are more complex and more accurately imitate the movements we perform in everyday life.

An easy way to integrate functional training into fitness training is to write down what your clients do every day, what their physical challenges are. Has your client noticed that her legs and back hurt at the end of her workday because she is constantly sorting binders and lifting them from the floor to her desk or placing them on shelves? Then that should be the first body region you work on. Examples of functional movements that use multiple joints and muscle chains are

❭ multidirectional lunges,
❭ standing bicep curls, and
❭ step-ups with weights.

Multidirectional lunges prepare the body for many different everyday activities, such as vacuuming or yard work. In doing so, the lunge is not just performed in a forward direction, but in many different directions at various angles. It is recommended to start with exercises that use only your own body weight for physical loading. Weights and resistance can be integrated into the exercises as the fitness level increases.

2.4 WHAT IS A FUNCTIONAL PERSONAL TRAINER?

Success can be defined in many different ways—as is true in personal training. I define success not by a full appointment book, but by the ability to make yourself indispensable as a fitness trainer, which has the paradoxical effect that your clients want more of you. Moreover, being successful means providing excellent service, especially to those who effectively need help. In times of burnout and back problems, excellent service on the body of humanity in an unsaturated market doubtlessly guarantees a constant inflow of clients for decades to come.

From my perspective, there are five key factors that make a successful trainer.

1. LEAD RATHER THAN FISH FOR APPLAUSE

A successful trainer instills in his clients the desire for physical fitness and the ability to achieve it, irrespective of his person. It is not about doing a "killer workout" with the client and then telling him good job, even if it isn't true. Lead someone to their personal fitness, meaning use their existing resources—like an internal hard drive—and steer them in the right direction, providing holistic instruction and not just workouts. Make yourself obsolete and something absurd happens: Your clients will become "addicted" to this special kind of fitness and thrive in a way you never thought possible. From then on, they will work out regularly and intensely (i.e., doing the "hard work"), but you get all the credit. That is because you helped the client find his own personal fitness and not just provided exercises. If you are able to change your clients' attitude about fitness in a positive way, their bodies will inevitably also change in a positive way.

2. DO AWAY WITH THE "CALORIES IN VS. CALORIES OUT" MYTH

The worst lies are the ones that contain more than just one grain of truth.

The laws of physics and thermodynamics make this myth appear to be a rock-solid finding, but the human individual is a self-aware being. This unremarkable psychological factor has serious effects on our biology and health. A study done at Yale University in 2011 in which people were given the same shake with differing information regarding calorie content (i.e., less than the actual content or more) provided an impossible result from a research point of view (lab). After consuming the "healthy" shake, the hormone ghrelin was suppressed only briefly and, thus, slightly, while the suppression of ghrelin after the "unhealthy" shake increased. Thus, the subjects that consumed the healthy shakes were hungry again sooner than the other subjects. Be aware of the power of the mind and the individuality of a human being!

3. TRAIN AND USE WHAT WORKS FOR YOUR CLIENT

Avoid being a "BOSU guy" or "kettlebell girl." Never define yourself purely by a piece of equipment you use. That does not mean that exercise equipment isn't an important and very useful addition to fitness training, but we will get to that later. Define yourself by your results! Training with a limited range of equipment or methods limits your ability and creativity and, thereby, the progress and satisfaction of your clients. Furthermore, not every piece of equipment is right for every client, even if just for reasons of personal preference. This is also true for available technology in the form of physical activity monitoring devices, pulse monitors, and smartphone apps, for example. Always use what will lead the client to achieve his individual goal in the quickest and simplest way. That work is already hard enough.

4. WORK ON MOVEMENT FIRST

Two facts from today's world: A large and growing number of people are overweight or even obese and suffer from other so-called lifestyle diseases, and the population as a whole is getting older. People must and want to feel better. They will choose the path that leads to increased well-being and improved mobility that makes it possible to handle everyday life and find pleasure in everyday things again. By helping our clients achieve this goal and providing a comprehensive training system that has an appropriate starting point for everyone's individual fitness level, we bring about a paradigm shift. This approach has enormous potential for our success for two reasons.

First of all, our future success depends on our ability to reach the "lifestyle-sick" and aging population. If we succeed, we have access to a growing and still largely untapped market. Until now, we have expected these people to come to us, but we must meet this target group in particular where they stand and accompany them individually.

Secondly, thanks to scientific research and many continuing education opportunities, the quality of knowledge transfer continues to increase. Today's student is tomorrow's trainer—the trainer with a more complex fundamental training unless we adapt our training methods to the current conditions and knowledge. In recent years, I have focused my training efforts on improving movement overall, and I have to say that, over time, one reaches a "faith healer-like" status among clients. You will experience many "I-can't-believe-it-doesn't-hurt!" moments, and as a result, more mouth-to-mouth recommendations than you can handle.

5. USE INTENSITY INTELLIGENTLY

Is it any wonder that the public often has a problem with the current glut of personal trainers in the fitness industry? Some trainers still think that vomiting after a hard workout, muscular acidosis, or bloody calluses are training effects to be celebrated. Injuries of any kind to one's body, regardless the type, are never a reason for celebration! Intensity without intelligence or knowledge is one of the biggest problems in every sector, including the fitness industry. Yes, intensity leads to results, but low, medium, or high intensity depends on someone's current personal fitness level. Trainers who sooner or later disappear from the industry are the types that pick up clients at their front door with an intense workout and measure success by the amount of pouring sweat. If you are this extreme stereotype of a trainer, you will probably also be the first budget cut when the client is short on cash. We can find "hard workouts" in nearly every fitness magazine, online videos, fitness websites, and books. They are a dime a dozen. But the ability to accompany someone through his personal athletic development, not only with compassion and strength, but also with the independence needed to build confidence in his athletic abilities, is what makes a true fitness professional—a fitness professional who has the ability to exist long-term in the industry.

In my opinion, next to these five key factors, a personal trainer should have the following characteristics:

1. COMPASSION AND AUTHENTICITY

You must love and live what you do. That is the only way to be credible and have the strength to trust and have faith in you.

2. EMPATHY AND UNDERSTANDING

Every person is wired differently. Find out what makes someone tick. What are his goals, dreams, fears, and limits? Understanding is the key to success. Work with the client's lifestyle and support him through his mental and physical changes, but always be aware that what is normal for you is not necessarily normal for your client!

3. THE WILLINGNESS TO KEEP LEARNING AND PUSH LIMITS

The software and hardware of the fitness industry is constantly changing, and as a fitness trainer, it is, therefore, important to always be up to date. It keeps you fresh and motivated and always provides the client with the latest fitness knowledge. Learn from exceptional trainers and choose people as teachers who will inspire you. Continuing education in business management, NLP, psychology, sports therapy, together with all my fitness knowledge gives me the unique opportunity to bring about change. In doing so, the key to success is to convey your complex knowledge to your clients in a readily understandable way.

4. THE ABILITY TO IDENTIFY NICHES AND UTILIZE THEM

Each person has special abilities and aptitudes. Use these niches to make a name for yourself and to specifically serve your clients with this knowledge. Moreover, this ability gives you the opportunity to share your knowledge with the broader public through articles in trade magazines, books, or as a convention speaker. It is a way to heighten your profile and boost your business skills.

5. THE ABILITY TO GIVE BACK

By holding charity events for a good cause, I raised £33,000.00 (approximately $47,000.00 USD) and brought new target groups to physical fitness. That is a fantastic feeling and reinforces your belief that you are doing the right thing.

6. WALK THE WALK

Achieving others' goals only works if you also accomplish your own goals, no matter how rocky the path. You are your own trademark. Live it! The way you live, work with your clients, and speak reflects who you are.

2.5 REQUIREMENTS FOR A SUCCESSFUL PERSONAL TRAINING BUSINESS

Recently someone asked me about the top 10 requirements for a successful personal training business. To be honest, at first I was not sure how to answer them. There are so many things that impact success, but the top 10? Here is my top 10 list for a successful personal trainer and, thus, business, compiled after much contemplation, but I would really like to hear your top 10 list!

TOP 1
Education
Professional and continuing.

TOP 2
Integrity
Consistency of your values and principles.
Without integrity, you are not credible and are a "nobody."

TOP 3
Experience
The more experience you have, the more customized the programs you design for your clients are. Experience allows you to be not only creative, but also effective in your interactions with clients and in creating the optimal environment.

TOP 4
Teaching methods
There are lots of people out there who are able to get their bodies in shape and may have the knowledge to be a top personal trainer. But if they aren't able to teach, their body and knowledge are of no use.

TOP 5
Communication
Good communication means good business, regardless of the industry. The ability to communicate brings clients to your training location and keeps them there.

TOP 6
Passion
For the client and the service you provide.

TOP 7
Organizational skills
Next to organizing the individual fitness programs of clients you must nurture client relations and coordinate their appointments. In addition, there are many operational matters that must be organized.

TOP 8
The ability to motivate
Get everyone to do his or her best. Take them out of their comfort zone, and do so regularly. That doesn't happen without motivation (at least in the beginning).

TOP 9
Work ethic
A great work ethic makes a good trainer into a professional trainer.

TOP 10
Natural helper
Good trainers love to help others. Satisfaction as the payoff for clients reaching their goals is one of the greatest assets of a professional trainer.

And there are certainly other important characteristics a professional trainer should possess, because a perfect fitness pro wears many hats.

CHAPTER 3

TRAINING CONTENT

3

TRAINING CONTENT

3.1 THE FOUR PILLARS OF HUMAN MOVEMENT

When taking an objective look at human movement we are able to describe our natural functions in a very simple way. These are our body's natural tasks—the way it moves, its use, and its functions. When your are familiar with the body's functions, it is easy to figure out what functional training should look like.

FIRST PILLAR: STANDING AND MOVING

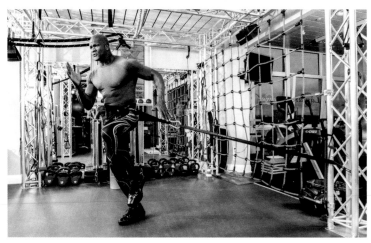

Photo 1

44

The first pillar of our movement is standing and moving, whereby we can shift our center of gravity linearly.

SECOND PILLAR: CHANGING THE PLANE OF THE CENTER OF GRAVITY

The process of changing planes is important here. Plane changes are movements of the trunk and the lower extremities, or a combination of both processes, that raise or lower the body's center of gravity. In doing so, the degree of difficulty of the exercises can be increased at will with different body positions.

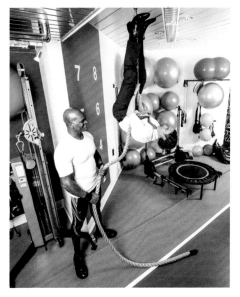

Photo 2

THIRD PILLAR: PULLING AND PUSHING

The third pillar of human movement is pulling and pushing.

With these movements, we shift the body's equilibrium by using the upper body.

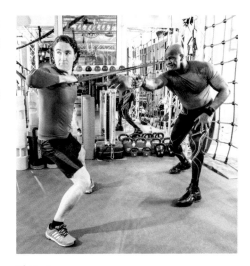

Photo 3

FOURTH PILLAR: ROTATION – DIRECTIONAL CHANGE AND TORQUE

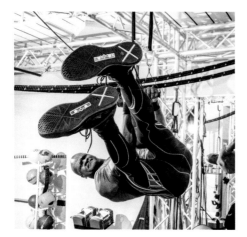

The brain's cross-wiring brings us to the most important pillar of human movement: directional change and torque. This pillar describes the part of the crisscrossing nerve endings of human movement.

Photo 4

3.2 THE THREE PLANES OF HUMAN MOVEMENT

We will now focus on the three-dimensional nature of our environment as another element of human movement. Knowing the positional and directional terms of the body and their significance in functional training is pivotal when choosing the right movements and designing effective training programs.

Table 3: Positional and directional terms

Ventral	On the abdomen
Dorsal	On the back
Lateral	To the side
Medial	To the middle
Cranial	Toward the head
Caudal	Downward
Proximal	Close to the body
Distal	Away from the body
Anterior	In the front
Posterior	In the back
Superior	Above
Inferior	Below
Ipsilateral	On the same side of the body
Contralateral	On the opposite side of the body
Plantar	The sole of the foot
Palmar	The palm

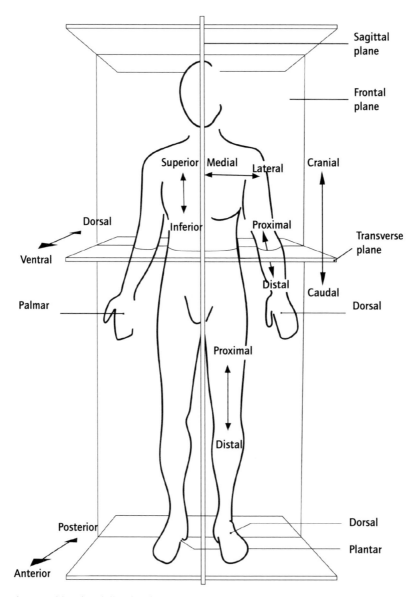

Fig. 5: Positional and directional terms and planes

Depending on the type of joint, one or several of the following basic movements shown in table 4 can be performed.

Table 4: Basic joint movements

Flexion	Bending
Extension	Straightening
Abduction	Outward movement away from the center of the body or a limb
Adduction	Inward movement toward the center of the body or a limb
Anteversion	Front raise (arms or legs)
Retroversion	Back raise
Protraction	Pushing forward (e.g., the scapula)
Retraction	Pulling back
Elevation	Lifting above a horizontal line
Depression	Lowering below a horizontal line
Rotation	Turning (internal and external)
Supination/pronation	Turning (hand/foot)

In fitness training, normal joint function (integrity) and mobility is an important basis for normal proprioception and reflexive stabilization. The capsular mechanoreceptors must transmit the right information (e.g., joint position) to be able to regulate motor function.

Each day, we move in an environment that allows us 360 degrees for possible movements. Conforming to the three-dimensional nature of our surroundings, we can divide it into three planes of movement. The vertical (sagittal plane), the frontal plane, and the horizontal (transverse) plane are the planes on which we move.

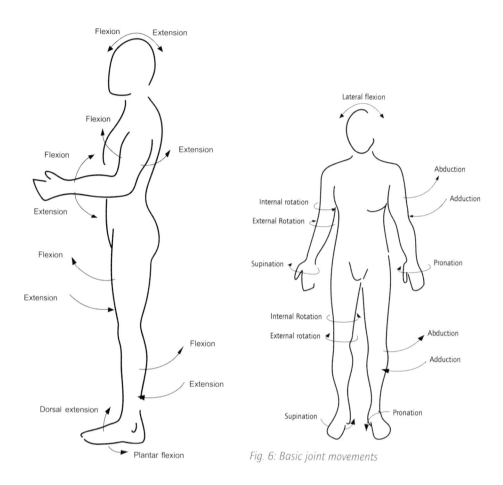

Fig. 6: Basic joint movements

The body's anatomical position is standing upright, face forward, arms at sides, palms facing forward, and fingers and thumbs extended. The definitions and descriptions of the body's planes and axes apply to this position. The vertical plane divides us into a right and left side, the frontal plane separates front from back, and the horizontal plane is the rotational plane that separates top from bottom.

The vertical plane (sagittal)	– Right and left half
The frontal plane	– Front and back section
The horizontal plane	– Upper and lower section

Although these three planes differ, human movement includes all planes, and most of our movements take place on multiple planes. Even when thinking of movements that initially just take place on one plane, it is possible to add other planes by moving the limbs. This idea offers various training options and progressions that we will look at more closely in chapter 5.

3.3 ENVIRONMENT

The four pillars provide a powerful basis for the design and integration of specific exercises into training. We can only improve training and, thereby, the performance of the trainee when we have a basic understanding of the environment of each individual we work with. We will, therefore, take a closer look at the environment.

3.3.1 GRAVITY OR WEIGHT

The human environment is defined by several basic parameters that we are all subject to and that we can adapt to. The most powerful and most constant parameter is gravity. It is existential and has a significant impact on our world. It is the force with which a body is pulled toward the earth.

Gravity dispenses resistance 24 hours a day and, thereby, enables the continuous remineralization of every living being's bones and the strengthening of muscles. Moreover, it helps us to use our muscles dynamically and to intensify or vary our muscle contractions. This is one of the reasons why we are able to perform a bigger lateral jump, for instance, when we can start with a preparatory counter movement instead of jumping from a static squat position. Gravity affects our activity by providing us with downward resistance (vector). This inertia component allows us to stand (or sit or lie) in one place until an external force changes that position. Gravity, thus, affects our weight while we move as well as the weight of external weights, such as free weights and other small equipment.

Gravity also affects our posture. Posture refers to the proper alignment of the parts of the body and, thereby, the joints under the effects of gravity. Posture is, therefore, a limiting factor in every movement. A correct posture protects joints and structures from damage and overloading and facilitates economical force transmission. Hence, creating a correct posture should be the foundation of every training program.

3.3.2 MASS, INERTIA, AND ACCELERATION (IMPULSE)

Various scientists and philosophers have provided detailed descriptions of the physical elements in our sphere of activity.

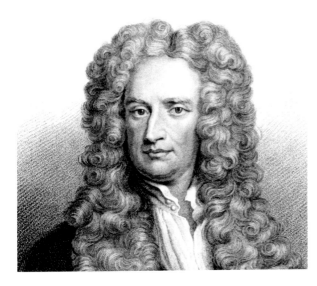

Fig. 7: Sir Isaac Newton (1642-1726)

Sir Isaac Newton used biomechanical processes to demonstrate what happens to objects under the influence or in the absence of forces—or how moving objects or objects that come into contact with each other behave and transfer their kinetic energy to each other. Transferred to human movement, this means that the following parameters always impact our fitness training:

❭ Physical effort under the influence of gravity (pushing something against a wall, blocking an opponent, lifting weights)
❭ Contact (punching, running into something)
❭ Starting/accelerating and decelerating/stopping (pursuit of opponents, serve/return play)

This means that Newton's basic assertions definitely enhance our knowledge regarding the function of the human body.

Newton's first law, the law of inertia, tells us that a body will remain at rest or in uniform motion in a straight line unless acted upon by an external force that changes its state. So if we want to function in our environment, we must overcome or disturb our body's state of inertia by standing up, swinging a golf club, or kicking a ball. Conversely, in fitness training, we can benefit from this law by causing an active disturbance. Is an athlete still able to perform a linear motion when he is subjected to lateral traction or must lift an additional weight?

The fundamental law of dynamics tells us that the acceleration (a) of a body as produced by a net force (f) is directly proportional to the magnitude of the net force in the same direction as the net force and inversely proportional to the mass of the object ($V = m \times a$ or mass x acceleration). The greater or more impulsive the acting force, the greater the acceleration, or the faster we run or the heavier we or the objects (e.g., balls, weights) are, the greater the resulting force.

Since mass is a constant, force can only be affected by speed. Here acceleration and deceleration should be considered equally as dynamic actions. The impact of force is never slow or controlled, nor does it take place on a single plane of movement.

Trendy products, such as tubes filled with pellets, sand or water, sacks, or clubs, that have been on the market since 2014 are wonderful toys for experiencing the power of dynamics and speed in training and, more importantly, to control it.

The law of action and reaction tells us that for every force acting on a body, the body exerts a force having equal magnitude and the moving opposite direction along the same line of action as the original force. We use this law every day when we pick up our children and brace our feet against the floor, or when we catapult ourselves out of the starting blocks for a sprint. This law, too, is a constant companion in dynamic training.

This basic biomechanical knowledge provides us with important information for effective training with our clients.

The goal of biomechanics is the description and analysis of motion sequences based on mechanical and biological knowledge. Mechanical properties of movement and the body are measured, and a qualitative description is given.

The results are transferred to the human biological system on the basis of mechanical laws with the goal of ascertaining the mechanical requirements of the act to be performed.

The resulting knowledge is critical to the evaluation of kinetic technique, methodological approach, and training devices.

Next to these basic laws, the following biomechanical concepts also play an important role in creating a training plan.

3.3.3 LEVER AND TORQUE

Muscle is a contractile organ that enables parts of the body to move against each other. These movements take place around pivot points or axes. This fact is very important to the implementation of force because these rotations of parts of the body and joints constantly create different torques or lever ratios that require a constantly changing muscular effort. The musculature adapts to the conditions to ensure a consistent motion sequence. So if a force (f) is applied to a pivot point at a distance (i) from the pivot point (moment arm), the torque (m) is defined as the product of force and distance of force to the point where force is applied: $m = f \times l$ (Nm) or torque = force x lever.

This means that the same amount of torque can be achieved with a longer lever and less force or with a shorter lever and more force. What is "saved" in force must be added in distance (level) or vice versa. An important factor in choosing exercises!

Biomechanics, and especially torque, also play an important role in the use of elastic resistance devices such as tubes and elastic bands. Here torque is affected by another factor, the force angle. The force angle is the angle that results from force and lever arm. It increases in proportion to the joint angle.

The muscle is weakest at the end point of the range of motion. For that reason, only a small force angle is required. Here the appropriate use of resistance can create optimal training conditions.

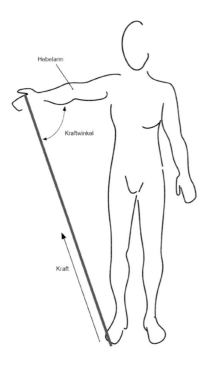

Fig. 8a: Torque and force angle

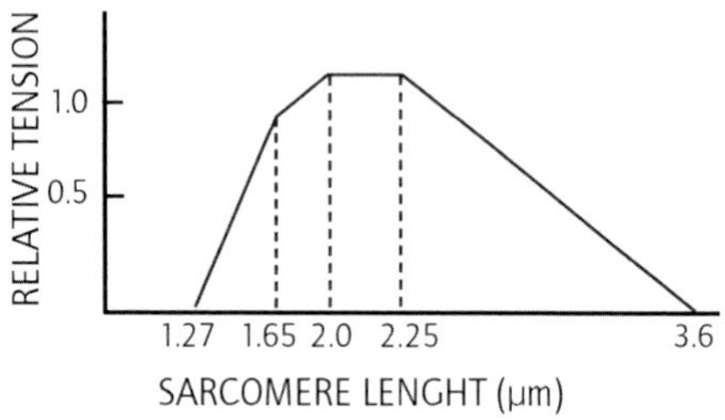

Fig. 8b: Muscular strength curve

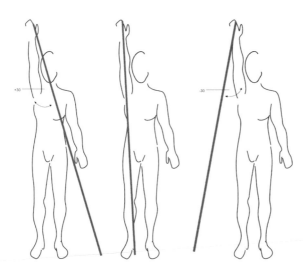

Fig. 8c: Band position for optimal strength utilization

For optimal strength utilization, the origin of the elastic resistance should be on the same line as the rotational axis (fig. 8c, center). Only then is a low force action at the beginning and the end of a movement guaranteed, which is particularly important in physical therapy and rehabilitation.

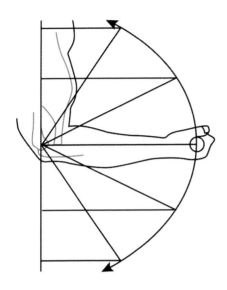

Fig. 9: Range of motion

In summary, considering the correct increase in resistance with clients in the beginning stages is important. As long as you work with basic exercises (chapter 5.1) and focus on facilitating movements and adjusting muscular imbalances, you should absolutely take this knowledge into account. In complex functional training for increased fitness, this knowledge can take a backseat since the client then has enough strength and stability in his movement patterns to tolerate a higher strength effort with extreme joint positions.

Thus, biomechanics deal with those factors that are important for the trainer and physical therapist in their daily practice.

❱ Which biomechanical factors does the performance depend on?

❱ How can the performance be improved?

❱ How can physical qualifications be improved?

❱ Which factors impact the strain on the movement apparatus?

❱ How can damages from overloading and incorrect loading be avoided?

❱ What role does training equipment play here?

3.4 STRENGTH AND CORE STABILITY – SUITABLE EXERCISES AND TESTS

Many daily activities require the use of multiple joints and take place on different planes. They are dynamic movement patterns that require a transfer of force between the extremities. Here the trunk occupies a key position in the transfer of force.

A weak, out-of-shape trunk increases the risk of injury to the lower back region during dynamic and ballistic exercises. In contrast, a fit trunk

> increases the effectiveness of movements;
> improves muscle balance and coordination;
> improves posture and gait;
> increases strength and flexibility in the lumbar and pelvic areas, as well as the sacroiliac joint (SIJ); and
> minimizes loss of energy and improves the transfer of force.

A mistake made time and again in training design is starting with strength training before ensuring sufficient trunk stability through exercises. This is comparable to the construction of a house where the foundation is reinforced only after several stories have already been built.

Posture exercises, stretches, and basic trunk stabilization exercises are important and should be at the top of every training program.

3.4.1 STRUCTURE (EXERCISE EXAMPLES)

PHASE ONE – TRUNK STABILIZATION
Movements are characterized by few repetitions; low, reduced intensity; and a progressively longer duration.

Goal: Internal stabilization, improved neuromuscular control.

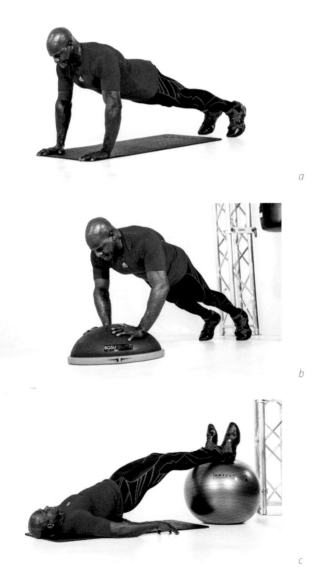

a

b

c

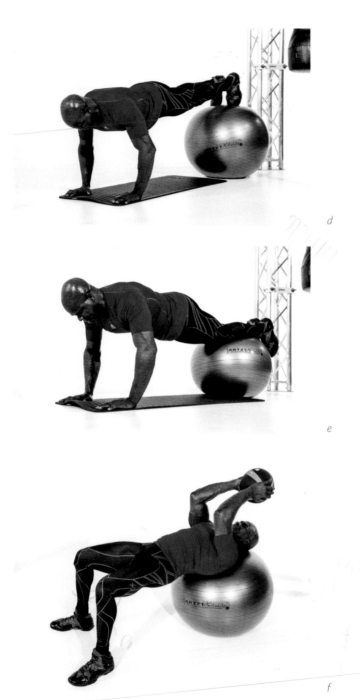

d

e

f

Photo 5 a-f: Exercise examples

PHASE TWO – TRUNK STRENGHTENING

Movements are more dynamic. Special ROM exercises on all planes of movement are used in contrast to body weight or external resistance.

Goal: Strengthen muscles and integrate movements.

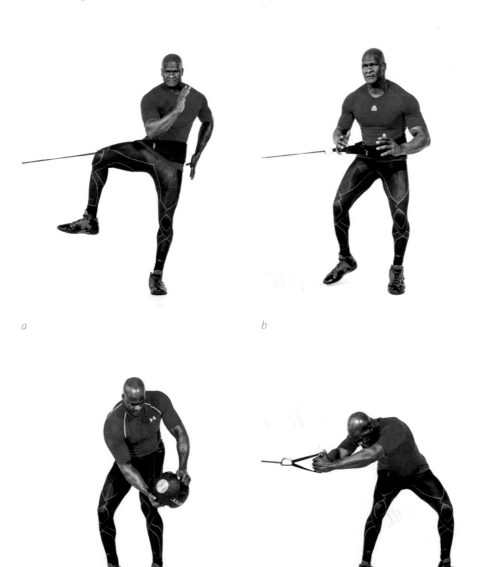

a

b

c

d

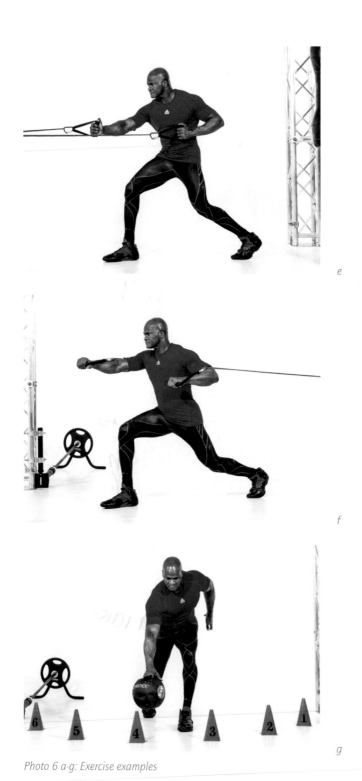

e

f

g

Photo 6 a-g: Exercise examples

PHASE THREE – TRUNK STRENGTH

Forces are generated and transferred into real time.

Goal: Replicating daily activities.

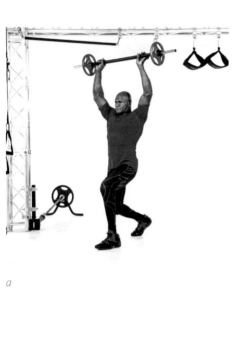

a

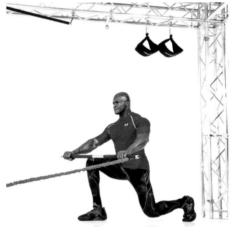

b

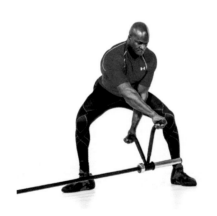

c

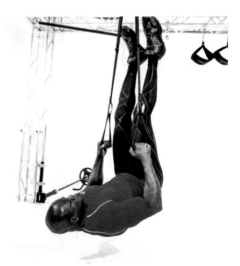

d

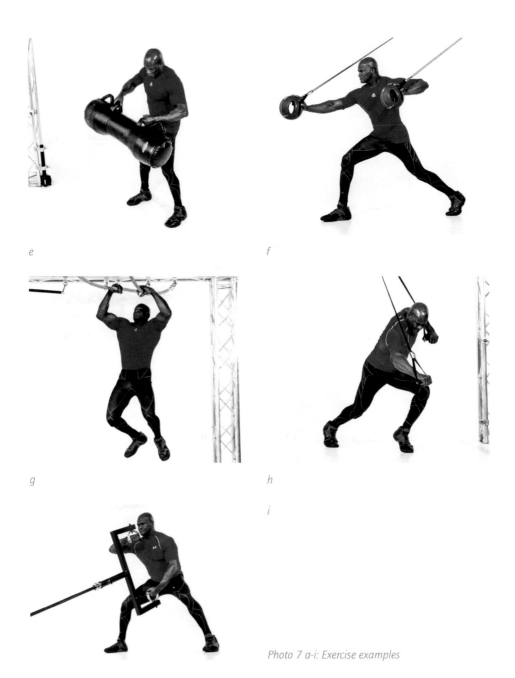

e

f

g

h

i

Photo 7 a-i: Exercise examples

But even with good basic strength, other parameters play a role in achieving a good fitness level. If a good fitness level were to be measured strictly by a person's ability to hold a position steady, professional bodybuilders would be the best athletes in the world. Maintaining trunk stability in a static position is but one step on the path to balanced trunk stability and a good physical fitness level. An important step nevertheless, but not the only one. Mobility is another key factor, and you can test it the following way.

When performing an exercise, are you able to maintain trunk stability when a certain amount of mobility of the joints in your upper and lower extremities is required at the same time? The best way to test this is with an Olympic lift. During this exercise, the weight is held overhead. Begin by standing with your arms extended and your trunk upright. During the subsequent squat, the arms remain extended and the upper body upright. What happens when the upper body cannot be kept upright is obvious. Joint mobility above and below the trunk is a limiting factor here. It restricts the range of motion and does not permit an optimal and for the body economical movement execution.

Non-strength athletes can do this exercise very well without a weight, using a bar or a broomstick. To do so, stand close to a wall, face the wall, and try to do a squat without falling backward. Often the wall already stops the movement during the beginning phase, or a lack of mobility in the hips and ankles prevents you from moving into a deep position.

3.4.2 LOWER BODY STRENGTH

Strength and performance are two different things. While strength means the ability of muscles to exert a lot of force, power is the ability to generate a force in very little time. But in reality, the two are closely linked. Top athletes work on both: They lift heavy weights to build more strength, and they move lighter objects at a high rate of speed to work on power. This allows them to move quickly (expression of their power) and to hit hard. The deadlift is probably the best indicator of your basic strength because it is comparable to many daily tasks, such as lifting or pushing heavy boxes or furniture.

This exercise works on the muscle strength of the back of the body: hamstring, gluteals, erector spinae, and trapezius.

You need these muscles to walk and jump or to bear up against someone who wants to knock you over. Moreover, they are among the largest muscles that also grow the fastest, so deadlifts definitely help to build muscle mass.

Attach weights to a barbell and place it on the floor. Your feet are shoulder-width apart and your toes point forward. Bend your hips and knees and grip the bar with an overhand grip just to the outside of your legs and pull it up to shin level. Now push your hips back, straighten your legs, and tighten your entire body from your feet all the way to your hands. Pull the barbell straight up until you stand upright and the bar is in front of your thighs. Then lower it back to the floor, keeping it as close to the body as possible. To warm up, start with a low weight and add more weight with each lift until you have reached your maximum weight.

3.4.3 LOWER BODY STRENGTH PLUS PERFORMANCE

There are few sports in which the feet always remain on the ground. Most require jumping and running. Doing so requires pushing off with one or both legs to achieve a maximum height, width, and speed.

The vertical leap is one of the most common methods for determining lower body performance capacity. However, the standing long jump is easier to measure since it does not require special equipment. The long jump is the easiest way to test the ability to combine force and power in one movement.

Stand with your toes behind a line on the floor. Your feet are a little less than shoulder-width apart. Get into a crouch and at the same time swing your arms backward. Now jump as far as possible while swinging your arms forward. You must land on both feet or the jump is invalid. It is best to do a few test jumps to get a feel for the movement, and then go all out. Mark the spot where your heels touch down (if you land with one foot slightly ahead of the other, you must mark the shorter distance), and then make a few more attempts. Finally, measure your best jumping distance.

3.4.4 THE WHOLE BODY

The bench press is the best exercise for building muscles and strength in the chest area. However, basic push-ups work more muscles even if not all of them are worked at maximum intensity. Like the bench press, push-ups work chest, shoulders, and triceps to exhaustion. The muscles of the abdomen, hips, and lower back also participate because they must maintain a stable spinal position. The greatest advantage of push-ups is probably that they work the muscles around the shoulder blades since these muscles support the shoulder joints. By comparison, the bench press can be very one-sided when the movement is always performed in one position.

3.4.5 UPPER BODY STRENGTH

Get into push-up position with your hands positioned directly below your shoulders, your feet hip-width apart and your weight on your hands and toes only. Your body must form a straight line from neck to ankles. Now lower your body until your chest is just a couple inches above the floor. Hold this position for a second (very important) and then return to your starting position. Do as many repetitions as you can with proper form.

Just like the bench press has replaced the push-up in many training programs, the pull-up had to make way to the lat pulldown. It really is a shame. Both exercises use the muscles of the upper and middle back—the latissimus dorsi, the lower trapezius, and the posterior deltoid—but the pull-up works additional muscles. Since you are hanging from a bar instead of sitting on a cushioned seat, the muscles of the middle back must work in tandem with those of the hips and lower back to maintain a stable spinal position. Pull-ups are well suited for tests. Lat pulldowns are certainly easier, but that's life. Nothing comes from nothing.

3.5 ENDURANCE

No movement is more important to survival than running. Still, many people misunderstand this. Most of us know that jogging is an aerobic activity. That means the body provides the energy it needs to move using oxygen. By contrast, sprinting is an anaerobic activity. One moves so fast that the muscles are unable to use oxygen and must, therefore, draw on other substances for energy. But running is also a test for muscular endurance. A 1000-meter run tests both areas. You need aerobic fitness to complete the distance at a decent time, and your muscles must be fit so your legs can bear up.

3.5.1 ENDURANCE AND FUNCTIONALITY

Many sports, such as tennis, basketball, team handball, volleyball, squash, badminton, and soccer, require a combination of lots of endurance, functionality, and strength.

Movements often become imprecise or uncontrolled when fatigue or even exhaustion sets in. This does not only cause the athletic performance to diminish, but also increases the risk of injury.

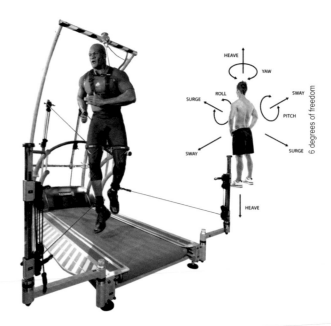

Photo 8: High-performance treadmill h/p/cosmos pulsar 3p with robowalk/roborun expander

Special treadmills such as the h/p/cosmos pulsar 3p make it possible to simulate and train these movements perfectly and safely using robowalk and roborun. For this purpose, a treadmill must be powerful and have a three-phase drive and have a running surface of at least 190/65 centimeters and extra-wide and anti-skid tread, so the user can quickly and safely jump off and on sideways during exercises. Robowalk makes it possible to simulate concentric, eccentric, and lateral loading stimuli.

That chapter is so complex and large that we can only briefly go into it in this book.

3.6 JOINT STABILIZATION, BALANCE, AND POSTURAL CONTROL

A FEW DEFINITIONS

Joint stabilization refers to the ability of joints (agonists and antagonists) to contract in order to support joints that are not moving during a movement and hold them in place. When this position has been achieved, we call it balance.

In kinematics and exercise science, balance is the ability to "maintain an upright posture against the forces of gravity and other disturbances while moving (dynamic balance)" (Pfeifer et al., 2001, p 262).

Von Pollock et al. define postural control as "the act of maintaining, achieving or restoring a state of balance during any posture or activity" (2000, p 402).

Many daily activities include dynamic movement patterns that use multiple joints on different planes and require the transfer of force between extremities. Joint stability, postural control, and balance play an important role here. Trainers should, therefore, emphasize this aspect of training because many exercises that are intended to provide people with more functionality require stability while generating force.

Stabilization training is a form of training in which force is limited by the structures necessary for stabilization as these cannot be utilized for the execution of the movement. This form of training can be performed either on an unstable surface, such as a stability ball, balance board, or balance pad, or with a smaller support surface, like doing one-leg instead of two-leg squats. In doing so, the progression should be as follows:

1. First with support, then without support or destabilized.

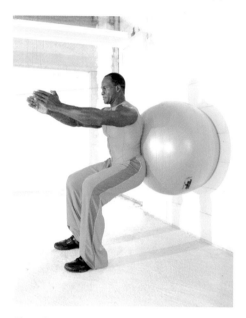

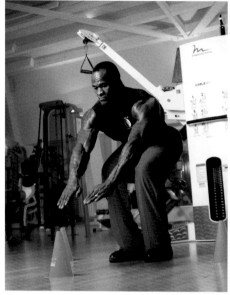

Photo 9

Photo 10

2. First bilaterally, then unilaterally.

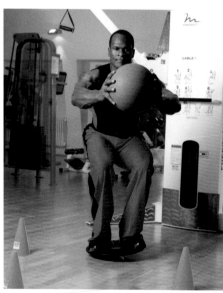

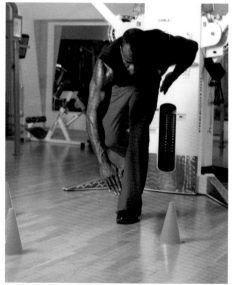

Photo 11

Photo 12

3. First a fixed lever, then a freely moving level.

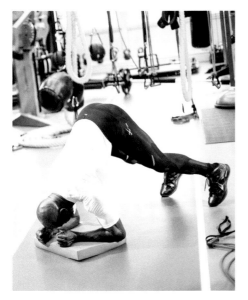

Photo 13

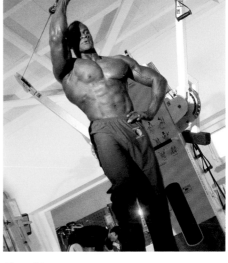

Photo 14

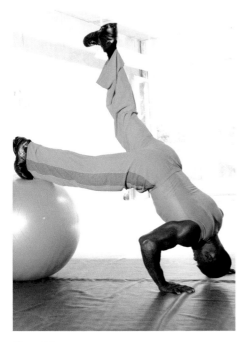

Photo 15

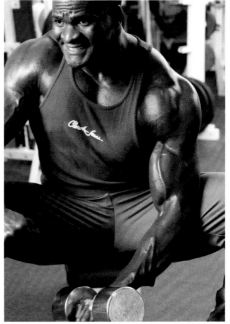

Photo 16

During such a functional movement, propulsive power can only transfer the force that trunk and stabilizers are able to support. This form of training can also be used effectively to improve the integrity of the trunk and other stabilizers that often impair the generation of force and power. This approach results in increased neuromuscular efficiency and improved transfer of force and joint stability because it promotes the integrity of the many joints that participate in the movement.

Stabilization training is a part of functional training. In addition, it can be easily combined with traditional fitness training. It is a good way to exhaust a part of the body in advance. For instance, you can first do a barbell press on a stability ball, followed by an incline bench press. In doing so, you work on stability as well as promoting muscle growth since the muscles are getting a sufficiently large stimulus from the traditional training.

3.7 PROPRIOCEPTION

Success depends on the synergistic function of the neuromuscular pathways, which is why it makes sense to work on the following: balance, proprioception, and force control.

The term proprioception stems from the Latin words (re)ceptus (to receive) and proprius (one's own) and is described by Sherrington as "the ability to perceive the condition and changing of joint angles via specific sensors" (Sherrington, 1947; Dickson, 1975; cited by Haas et al., 2006a, p 107). Perception or cognition with respect to your own body (proprio) is also called proprioceptive sensibility. In psychology, cognition is considered a holistic process—the entirety of information processing, from receiving (external and internal stimuli through receptors) to choosing and interpreting, all the way to organizing it. Special receptors in muscles, joints, and connective tissue help the body to receive information, process it, and react to it.

Proprioception is an automatic, endogenous, and, especially, sensitive mechanism that, simply put, sends information through the central nervous system. The central nervous system or its superordinate structures then transmit information and trigger a reaction (neuromuscular response), such as increased muscle tension. People do proprioceptive training to be able to perform everyday movements efficiently. Proprioception is largely automatic. In training, the goal is to make the perception of movements more conscious through mindfulness. Ideally this is done by

❯ double-tasking (peripheral focus),
❯ applying disturbance stimuli,
❯ varying the training stimuli,
❯ using ballistic, reactive movement patterns,
❯ removing sensory information (e.g., closing eyes), and
❯ limiting anticipation of the training situation.

This is an example to that end: You lift a 15-pound medicine ball with both hands and repeat this movement 10 times. Next you pick up a medicine ball that is lighter, but looks identical. You will notice that the body assumes the same amount of tension because it anticipates the same amount of weight as before. This is the result of a direct proprioceptive experience. The body's memory predetermines a certain exertion, but in this case does not require it.

Conscious perception and cognitive processing (e.g., the position of the body in space) can train neuromuscular control. Skin, palms, the soles of the feet, and other senses work together and communicate with the brain about muscle tension, shifting weight, and range of motion. Every functional exercise in which the body's center of gravity is held above the support surface helps to train the receptors in the entire body and, thus, train proprioception. Activities that require balance, coordination, mobility, and power and movements that make the client move beyond his usual range of motion are good tools for training proprioceptive adaptation.

One final example from that area: When someone trips and is unable to quickly regain his balance, it could be that the processes in the body are too slow to quickly react to the loss of balance—tripping. This person's proprioceptive ability can be trained by making the body react more quickly. The purpose of this type of training is to shorten the amount of time it takes for a physical reaction to take place and to also physically implement this task. The ability to move more quickly and powerfully effects a more precise transfer of instructions by the nervous system to the required muscles. This allows the body to react more quickly and accurately.

The following exercises and body systems have an effect on proprioceptive reaction:

❱ Movements with different patterns and ranges as well as degrees of muscle tension and loading (e.g., dancing, yoga, ballet, jumping rope, contralateral marching).
❱ Traditional endurance, strength, and mobility training.
❱ Balance exercises with open and closed eyes.
❱ Rotational movements (e.g., diagonal, horizontal, up and down, crisscross).
❱ Visual accuracy—using your visual sense to restore your balance; instead of looking down, keep your eyes forward.
❱ Hearing: The inner ear registers head and body movement like a built-in water level. For this to function properly, head and neck must be stacked above a balanced spine.
❱ Rhythm: Heartbeat, respiration, and even walking follow a natural rhythm. Every person should try to feel a rhythm when engaging in sports and performing movements.
❱ Stance: Movements should be performed from an athletic stance (ankles, knees, and hips slightly bent).

3.8   SMALL EQUIPMENT

Training trends and small equipment quickly come and go, but which ones are here to stay? Which of the touted pieces of small exercise equipment are truly effective and helpful to your clients? A piece of exercise equipment is only effective when its use is taught properly and individually. Much like the training plan, it must be consciously chosen for the respective individual. You can design the optimal training for your clients with their individual problems and diagnoses and decide which product is effective, providing you have first actively familiarized yourself with the equipment. Small exercise equipment often appears toy-like and, therefore, can create quick access to clients in a friendly way. Only what is fun will be continued long term. Small equipment can provide new motivation to you and your clients and facilitate the intensification and modification of exercises. With the targeted use of small exercise equipment you can

❱   prevent compensation,
❱   perform corrective exercises,
❱   apply new stimuli,
❱   increase functional requirements, and
❱   generate diversity and creativity.

My favorite pieces of exercise equipment are elastic resistance equipment (bands, loops, tubes), weights, ropes, and unstable surfaces.

3.8.1 ELASTIC RESISTANCE

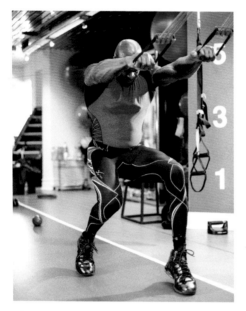

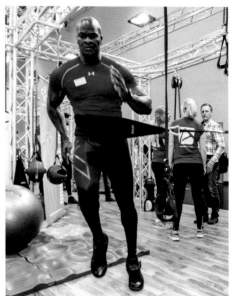

Photo 17

Photo 18

To date, bands have been greatly underrated as tools for functional training. Their apparently limited application in the area of rehabilitation is not representative of their true potential. For instance, running in place against resistance is an enhancement to power training as well as an aerobic program. In coordination and strength training you can choose the intensity for each client that is suitable for the respective training goal or target group. Few products are as versatile and flexible in their use as elastic resistance equipment. In addition, there are many case studies[1] that again prove that resistance training should not be absent from any functional training.

---

1 http://www.thera-bandacademy.com; http://www.gymstick.com/gymstick/gymstick/research.html

3.8.2 (FITNESS) BALLS AND WEIGHTS

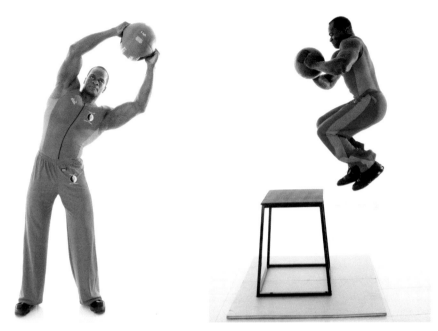

Photo 19   Photo 20

Modern medicine balls are made of rubber, come in different sizes and weights, and can have grips and built-in ropes. Since the whole body is used, the medicine ball can activate the entire kinetic chain. The balls can be used as weights to intensify any type of exercise. They can also be used to create an asymmetrical and unstable training environment. Only the trainer's imagination is the limit when designing a training program. I use the large fitness balls and the BOSU Balance Trainer as ideal training tools for balance and stabilization. Even if many of the exercises don't look like everyday movements, the stabilization requirements of these exercises are well suited for training important daily and sports patterns that are important for stability. The limiting factor in training with this type of small equipment is the right kind of stabilization and not the exertion of maximum strength.

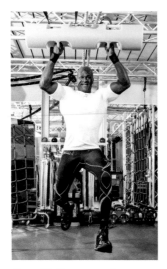

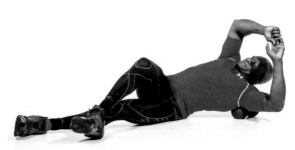

Photo 21: The power of water   *Photo 22: Myofascial release*

The industry constantly offers new toys to generate new motivation and new training stimuli.

When using small training equipment, your guiding principle should be: Individual tools for individual clients!

CHAPTER 4

STRUCTURE

4

STRUCTURE

Instead of looking at muscles separately, we now have a more complete image of movement patterns that show how movement is actually generated. This is not a difference pertaining to semantics, but rather taking into account the important role of the nervous system. According to the experts, intermuscular coordination (the way muscles work together to generate movement) that improves with function-oriented movement is of fundamental importance for improved general fitness. But we still don't know exactly what functional training means in practice and how to implement it.

Most trainers see movement patterns the following way:

> Squat
> Lunge
> Hip adduction
> Vertical press
> Vertical pull
> Horizontal press
> Horizontal pull
> Rotation
> Trunk flexion
> Trunk extension
> Trunk rotation

At first glance this appears to be a solid approach to strength training. But that's exactly the problem! We often only look at movements in terms of the weight room and not in terms of the demands we have to meet outside the weight room. The above movements are good. But they could be much better. The body is a complex system consisting of many chains. When these chains function properly they help us to move better and generate more power and speed. But if there is a weak link in the chain, we don't focus on the entire chain, but rather just the muscles and a very generic movement pattern.

4.1 THE PATH TO FUNCTIONAL PERFORMANCE

The reasons for a functional foundation have now been explained in detail. To achieve an optimal performance it is best to approach this goal step by step, as organized as possible. The first step focuses on analysis and determining which elements of performance are most important and which can be achieved the fastest. We can then estimate how much time this would take and how we can get good results as quickly as possible. This is especially important for personal trainers and physical therapists. A personal trainer may only have three or four appointments with a client. A physical therapist may have 6 to 12 appointments with a patient to figure out the problem. As personal trainers, we must, therefore, get quick results. We don't have the three to six months that are usually needed to build up muscle or correct muscular imbalances.

An important first step is the production of neuromuscular energy. The best way to stimulate a client's neurological system is through balance and coordination exercises. When a client does strength training, his strength increases, and the neurological elements have already been well developed. Because a trainer aims for neurological efficiency, he should tackle the problem as quickly and safely as possible and work on and stimulate the client's ability to stabilize positions he has not previously stabilized. As mentioned, human movement consists of four pillars, so the client must first learn these four basic skills.

Imagine the client is a child learning to walk. He has tried to do so for weeks and months. In the beginning, he needs support and holds on to a wall or a door.

Then he can slowly take his first steps. As the child gains confidence, the steps become steadier until he can finally walk. What happened? Did the client feel a change? Did he get stronger and was better able to perform the movements? The client didn't spend months following training plans, but his brain sent specific signals to certain muscles. These muscles then coordinated the movement the brain specified. After a few tries, the client was able to coordinate that movement.

That is exactly what happens with all other movements, from symmetrical or asymmetrical chest presses to bicep preacher curls with a barbell. The central nervous system sends signals, and eventually the muscles know what is expected of them. Finally the task is completed through a combination of increased recruiting (of utilized muscle fibers) and coordination (agonist and antagonist work together). So if you're short on time, building muscles is not the best method to make someone stronger in the least amount of time.

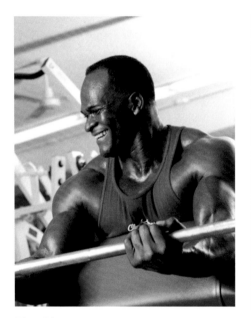 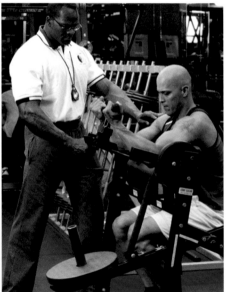

Photo 23   Photo 24

Another approach for training a client whose goal is improved function in everyday life is to further develop what is already there and to practice new things that could be of use to him. To do so, you begin with the four pillars and stabilization training.

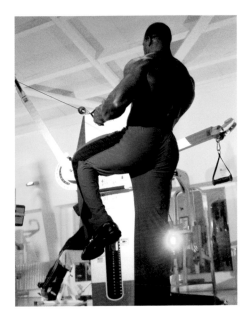

Photo 25

Regardless of age, anyone can learn skills like standing on one leg and reaching backward at their first appointment. This ability is immediately internalized and memorized, much like walking or riding a bike. As soon as that skill has been learned you hardly have to think about it. Just think how little practice walking or biking requires once you have learned it!

Stabilization and balance are natural aspects of skill development. The client learns to stabilize and balance in unusual but safe positions, which in turn trains his postural mechanisms and reflexes. Finally, it improves the client's ability to transfer force from the inside to the outside. These are natural processes the body uses to stabilize and protect itself. Training the four pillars isn't another form of physical therapy. With hard work and practice, functional training that teaches the aforementioned abilities can lead to unbelievable results with clearly recognizable progress.

The speed with which a force is generated is another important factor responsible for coordination. Sometimes speed can even be more important than the amount of force generated. The speed of force generation is the key element of performance and, like power, depends on the efficiency of the movement. This means that performance largely depends on neuromuscular efficiency. Functional training has a very big, positive impact on performance development.

Improving the neural factors by corresponding learning skills means a person can get stronger and do so not just by building muscle or training absolute strength. Showing the client how to better utilize natural, endogenous functional movements will allow him to reach his goal of achieving better health. We know that the body is able to release major forces even without physical training. For instance, in unexpected dangerous situations people are able to accomplish feats they ordinarily would not be able to. Each of us possesses practically supernatural strength, namely the ability to use the right muscles at the right time.

Over time, the client masters the four pillars. Structural changes take place. This is a natural process that does not have to be planned. Hans Selye's models of the general adaptation syndrome illustrate this: If a system is subject to increased stress, it reacts and adapts. Structural integrity can also consist of muscle development, but it can take several months, and in some people even years, before there are significant discernable results and changes. Thus, the question is, what happens when we work with someone who builds muscle mass very slowly? Does this mean any hope for structural integrity of his physiology is lost? There are different adaptations that will increase structural integrity without additional structures (muscle mass). For instance, increased structural integrity can be achieved through improved joint alignment. Improved joint alignment leads to increased balance and increased dexterity. All of this induces the efficacy of functional training with respect to neurological factors combined with dexterity.

Furthermore, it is important to continuously challenge your clients. Offer them challenges that keep training exciting. When the body is constantly placed in new positions, it is naturally aware of its surroundings. Movements are not necessarily planned. Success is based on stabilization, control, and testing and not on a particular number of repetitions and sets. Being frequently and suddenly confronted with challenging activities can be more effective in training body awareness than lengthy exercises. To do so, you place your clients in situations that promote their ability to assess positions and speed of movement relative to a fixed point, such as a hand or foot.

Thus, progression is a constant companion on the path to functional fitness because that is the only way you can constantly offer new stimuli. Progression is possible by

> decreasing the size of the support base,
> reducing points of contact,
> increasing endurance (static movements),

> transitioning from static to dynamic movement patterns,
> transitioning from simple to complex movement sequences,
> increasing repetitions (dynamic movements),
> switching from slow to fast, ballistic movement patterns (replicating everyday activities), and
> transitioning from low to higher force generation.

IN SUMMARY:

THE FUNCTIONAL PATH TO BETTER PERFORMANCE

Working on dexterity and the four pillars

1. INCREASE DEXTERITY
2. INCREASE STRENGTH
3. INCREASE POWER
4. INCREASE STRUCTURAL INTEGRITY
5. IMPROVE ALIGNMENT
6. IMPROVE BALANCE
7. LOWER BODY FAT PERCENTAGE

4.2 TRAINING ADAPTATION STEPS AND GUIDELINES

Those are the four steps and priorities of adaptation in fitness training. All components should be trained together and not one after the other.

TRAIN AS OFTEN AS POSSIBLE WITHOUT SUPPORT

That means the bulk of our resistance training should be done standing and not by supporting ourselves against an object. When you do all your training with support (i.e., while lying on a bench, sitting on a machine), you create a fairytale world for your body in which trunk stability and balance don't matter. Moreover, we have learned that while standing, athletes can only generate a third of the strength they generate when they bench press. So if you are able to bench press 550 pounds, it makes less sense to continue training in that anatomical position.

TRAIN PRIMARILY WITH FREE WEIGHTS

Training with free weights involves not only primary muscles, but also secondary muscles. Dumbbells, in particular, do not only improve strength, but also strength endurance, and due to their instability, promote muscle balance and an increased range of motion. This is in line with the previously mentioned effects of training without support.

TRAIN EXPLOSIVELY AS OFTEN AS POSSIBLE

Explosive weightlifting as it is done in the Olympics has many advantages. Even simple variations on classic Olympic weightlifting, like the clean, snatch, and jerk, can improve general strength, power, metabolism, and fitness—not to mention the positive effects on balance, range of motion, and mobility. Besides, moving loads quickly, regardless of how high they are, brings with it enormous advantages. These exercises train fast-twitch muscles, which is important in strength and power development.

COMPOUND EXERCISES

It is important to explain the reasons for doing multijoint compound exercises. Compound exercises are not only better for building strength, but also use more calories and induce a stronger endocrine reaction, which leads to increased growth hormone and testosterone levels. Thus, compound exercises increase the production of hormones that provide more strength. These exercises are also considerably more functional than exercises that activate only isolated muscles.

Another aspect of this training philosophy is the requirement that athletes press and pull on a vertical as well as horizontal plane, perform rotational movements, do exercises that focus on knees and hips, and perform all of these movements bilaterally (with two limbs) as well as unilaterally (with one limb).

Exercises should be presented individually, so the functional training method is used as previously indicated.

CHAPTER 5

PRACTICE

5

PRACTICE

Let me reiterate: The more closely the structure of a training exercise replicates an everyday or athletic movement sequence, the more effective the training result is! But in order for complex training exercises to really bring about positive effects and no damage, we must first create a good foundation. To facilitate efficient movement sequences and to improve movement control, we can also use isolating and supporting exercises. Here we proceed based on the principle: isolate – innervate – integrate – complex.

The first practice exercises are, thus, guided by basic therapeutic exercises that focus on individual muscle groups. In addition to the exercise descriptions, we list the primary and secondary muscles or muscle groups and provide a visual reference using a muscle anatomy diagram.

The second practice chapter offers complex exercises that can be done for the most part with small exercise equipment that boosts complexity and optimizes application in everyday life. Here emphasis is placed on the pillars and planes concept. And you can look forward to the "best of Lamar" exercises that will show you, and of course your clients, individual limits and options.

And for all the trainers among you who occasionally like to fall back on a predesigned workout, I put together seven workouts at the end of this chapter. In addition, some of the circuit trainings show the options an effectively equipped and thought-out training room like my PT (personal training) room can offer. Simple mounting options at various heights and angles as well as small equipment facilitate a diverse and fluid training process. Another plus for your functional trainer career.

As we begin to practice, there is, of course, the question of the best-possible training dosage. Most important here is your experience and the correct assessment of your client. Training dosage must be customized for your clients, their goals, and their habits, because that is the only way to make functional training successful long term.

My recommendations for this are as follows:

DOSAGE

1. A client assessment is necessary for a specific training dosage (assessment, see pg. 96).
2. Choose exercises that suit the client's personality, the sport he enjoys or his everyday demands, his training experience, your training equipment, and the client's availability.
3. Customize the training load for the client's individual fitness level, (sport) season, type of training, and his existing parallel demands in exercise and everyday life.
4. Exercises in one training unit should primarily be geared to the client, but also have a structured progression (i.e., coordination before strength, first without and then with equipment, from light to heavy).
5. To me, the simplest and most effective approach to recommending a training dosage is based on maximum load (repetition max) with regular intermediate checking.
6. Always gear load, number of repetitions, and sets to the training goals, the client's training condition, and the amount of available time.
7. Use progression in a sensible and timely manner.

POSSIBLE CLASSIFICATION OF CLIENTS

TRAINING STATUS
1. Beginner/beginner (unfit)
2. Recreational athlete/intermediate (moderately fit)
3. Athlete/advanced (fit)

CURRENT TRAINING WORKLOAD

1. None or less than two months of training experience (unfit)
2. Regular training for at least two months (moderately fit)
3. Frequent training for at least 12 months (fit)

TECHNICAL EXECUTION/MOVEMENT SKILLS

1. Low (unfit)
2. Moderate (moderately fit)
3. High quality (fit)

POSSIBLE TRAINING DOSAGE FOR FUNCTIONAL STRENGTH ENDURANCE TRAINING (BASIC TRAINING)

TRAINING FREQUENCY PER WEEK

1. 1-2 times/week (unfit)
2. 2-3 times/week (moderately fit)
3. 3-4 times/week (fit)

NUMBER OF REPETITIONS AND SETS

1. 8-10 reps, two sets (unfit)
2. 10-20 reps, three sets (moderately fit)
3. 20-30 reps, four sets (fit)

TRAINING LOAD

1. Low: 4 to 5 different exercises, vertical execution as well as a 5- to 10-minute anaerobic cardio component, performed in 1-minute intervals, such as jump rope or mini trampoline (unfit)
2. Mid-level/medium: 8 to 10 different exercises, executed on the vertical and frontal planes, as well as a 15- to 20-minute anaerobic cardio component performed in 1-minute intervals, explosive execution with power, such as jump rope, mini trampoline, jumping jacks, or burpees (moderately fit)
3. High: 10 to 15 different exercises, executed on the vertical, frontal, and transverse planes, as well as an approximate 20-minute anaerobic cardio component, performed in 1-minute intervals, explosive execution with powers, such as jump rope, mini trampoline, jumping jacks, or burpees (fit)

POSSIBLE DOSAGE FOR FUNCTIONAL STRENGTH TRAINING (INTERMIEDIATE TRAINING)

TRAINING FREQUENCY PER WEEK

1. 1-2 times/week (unfit)
2. 2-3 times/week (moderately fit)
3. 3-4 times/week (fit)

NUMBER OF REPETITIONS

1. 6-10 reps (unfit)
2. 6-10 reps (moderately fit)
3. 6-10 reps (fit)

TRAINING LOAD

1. Low: Three different exercises per muscle group. Large muscles: chest + small muscles: biceps. Weights must be individualized (2-22 lbs.).
2. Mid-level/medium: Five different exercises per muscle group. Large muscles: legs, biceps + small muscles: shoulders. Weights must be individualized (17-33/44 lbs.).
3. High: Eight different exercises per muscle group. Large muscles: back + small muscles: triceps. Weights must be individualized (22/44-55/110 lbs.).

The amount of weight depends on the client, the chosen body position, and the exercise angle, or rather, the acting lever.

The purpose of testing, or assessments, is the collection of a respective client's basis data that provides an objective foundation for designing exercise programs and determining training goals. The compilation and evaluation of different parameters provides you as the personal trainer with a more definite assessment of the client. Moreover, testing allows for better assessment of injury risk, an optimal introduction to training for the individual client, and the setting of realistic training goals (i.e., choice of exercises, dosage).

TIPS FOR COLLECTING BASIS DATA

There are many good reasons for doing assessments with your clients:

〉 Obtaining a baseline for future training progress or reasonable progressions
〉 Determining the current training condition or muscular imbalances or compensation patterns that might affect the planned training progress
〉 Compiling helpful data to determine intensity and volume of the exercises or the training program
〉 Using helpful data to determine short-, mid-, and long-term goals
〉 Identifying risk factors that would suggest a doctor visit might be prudent before the start of training
〉 Finding proof of the current condition that could be helpful in case of injury or illness after the start of training

Existing assessments can usually be completed with all clients and can be an additional source of income for trainers. But in doing so, you must make absolutely sure that tests do not take up too much time and the results are directly incorporated into program design. This should also be evident to your clients or else they might otherwise view the additional tests as a breach of confidence.

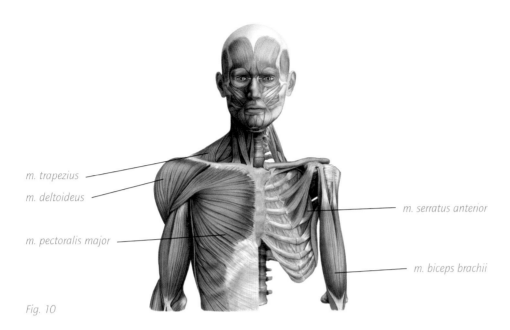

m. trapezius

m. deltoideus

m. pectoralis major

m. serratus anterior

m. biceps brachii

Fig. 10

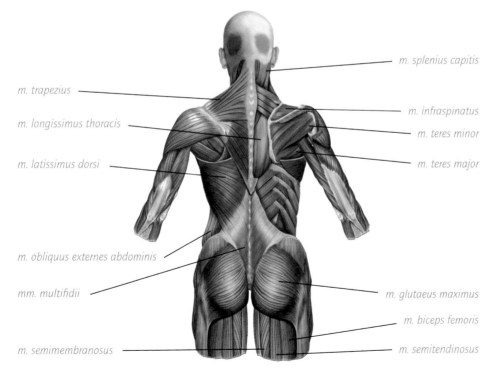

m. splenius capitis

m. trapezius

m. longissimus thoracis

m. latissimus dorsi

m. infraspinatus

m. teres minor

m. teres major

m. obliquus externes abdominis

mm. multifidii

m. glutaeus maximus

m. biceps femoris

m. semimembranosus

m. semitendinosus

Fig. 11

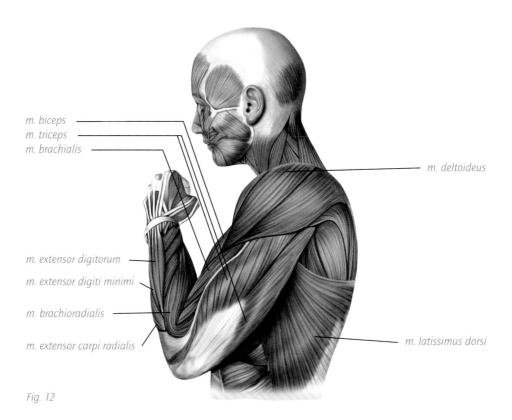

m. biceps

m. triceps

m. brachialis

m. deltoideus

m. extensor digitorum

m. extensor digiti minimi

m. brachioradialis

m. extensor carpi radialis

m. latissimus dorsi

Fig. 12

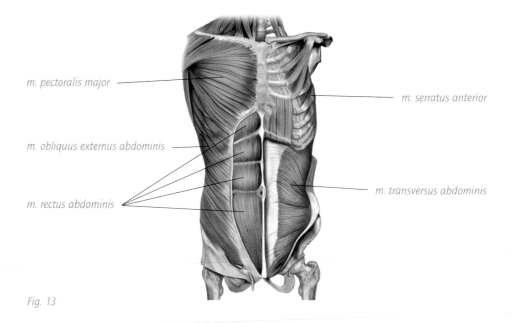

m. pectoralis major

m. serratus anterior

m. obliquus externus abdominis

m. rectus abdominis

m. transversus abdominis

Fig. 13

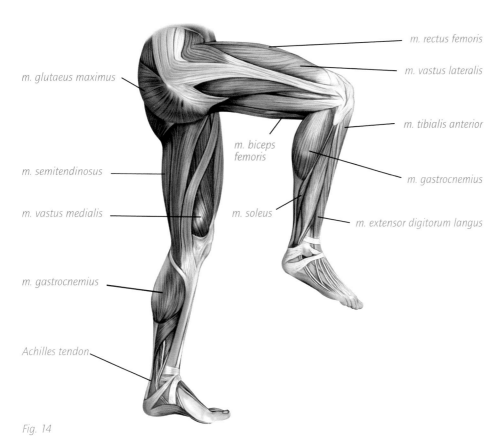

m. rectus femoris

m. vastus lateralis

m. glutaeus maximus

m. tibialis anterior

m. biceps
femoris

m. semitendinosus

m. gastrocnemius

m. vastus medialis

m. soleus

m. extensor digitorum langus

m. gastrocnemius

Achilles tendon

Fig. 14

Fig. 10-14: Superficial and deep musculature

5.1   THE BASICS

CHEST/BACK

M. LONGISSIMUS THORACIS – LONG CHEST MUSCLE

HYPEREXTENSION, LEG EXTENSION WITH LARGE FITNESS BALL

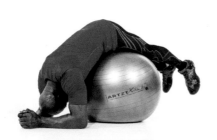
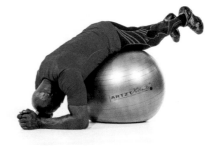

a

b

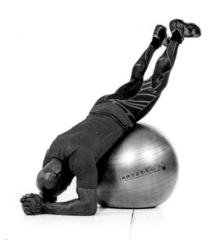

c

Photos 26 a-c

STARTING POSITION

You start on your abdomen. The ball is under your pelvic area. Support yourself on the floor with your forearms to help you keep your balance.

EXECUTION

Raise both legs until your thighs no longer touch the ball but your back is straight (don't arch your back). As you raise your legs, shift your weight to your forearms to keep your balance. Hold, and then return to the starting position.

PARTICIPATING MUSCLES

PRIMARY
Iliocostalis muscle (m. iliocostalis)
Long chest muscle (m. longissimus thoracis)
Multifidus muscle (mm. multifidii)

SECONDARY
Gastrocnemius, lateral head (m. gastrocnemius, caput laterale)
Gastrocnemius, medial head (m. gastrocnemius, caput mediale)
Large gluteal muscle (m. gluteus maximus)
Medium gluteal muscle (m. gluteus medius)
Semitendinosus muscle (m. semitendinosus)
Biceps femoris muscle (m. biceps femoris)
Semimembranosus muscle (m. semimembranosus)
Soleus muscle, calf (m. soleus)

MM. MULTIFIDII – MULTIFIDUS MUSCLE

SUPERMAN, ALTERNATING SIDES

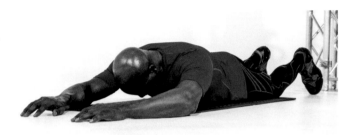

a

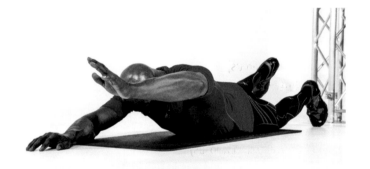

b

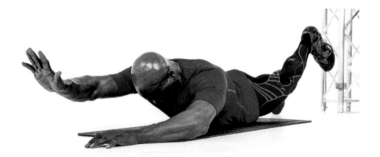

c

Photos 27 a-c

STARTING POSITION

Lie flat on your abdomen.

EXECUTION

Simultaneously lift one arm and the opposite leg.

PARTICPATING MUSCLES

PRIMARY

Iliocostalis muscle (m. iliocostalis)
Long chest muscle (m. longissimus thoracis)
Multifidus muscle (mm. multifidii)

SECONDARY

Large gluteal muscle (m. gluteus maximus)
Medium gluteal muscle (m. gluteus medius)
Semitendinosus muscle (m. semitendinosus)
Biceps femoris muscle (m. biceps femoris)
Semimembranosus muscle (m. semimembranosus)

MM. MULTIFIDII – MULTIFIDUS MUSCLE

HYPEREXTENSION WITH MEDICINE BALL

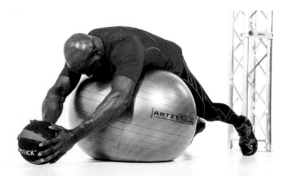

a

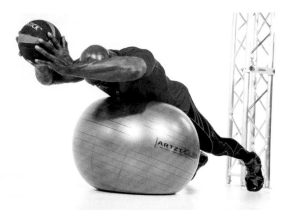

b

Photos 28 a-b

STARTING POSITION

Start with your abdomen on the large fitness ball. Rest your upper arms on the fitness ball. Legs are extended and toes touch the floor.

EXECUTION

Slightly lift your upper body off the ball and simultaneously raise your arms and the medicine ball to shoulder level. Then return to the starting position.

PARTICIPATING MUSCLES

PRIMARY
Iliocostalis muscle (m. iliocostalis)
Long chest muscle (m. longissimus thoracis)
Multifidus muscle (mm. multifidii)

SECONDARY
Straight abdominal muscle (m. rectus abdominis)

SHOULDERS, NECK, AND UPPER BACK

M. SPLENIUS – SPLENIUS MUSCLE GROUP

NECK STRETCHES WITH ADDED WEIGHT

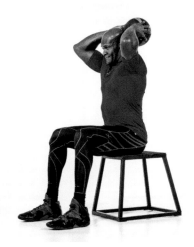

a

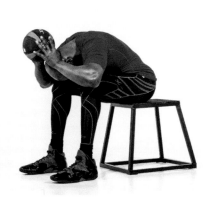

b

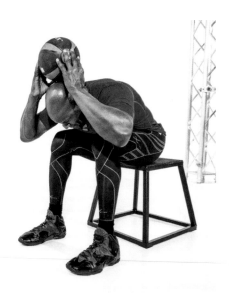

c

Photos 29 a-c

STARTING POSITION

Sit on a stool and place a weighted ball against the back of your head. Bend forward at the waist and hold the ball against the back of your head with both hands.

EXECUTION

Move your head backward by extending the cervical spine as much as possible. Now bend the cervical spine forward again until your chin touches your chest. Repeat.

PLEASE NOTE:
You can also use a barbell plate (place a towel underneath) instead of a weighted ball. To keep the load more even during the movement, the weight can move slightly during the head motion.

PARTICIPATING MUSCLES

PRIMARY
Splenius muscle of the head (m. splenius capitis)
Splenius muscle of the neck (m. splenius cervicis)

SECONDARY
Upper trapezius muscle (m. trapezius, pars descenders)
Levator scapulae muscle (m. levator scapulae)
Sternocleidomastoid muscle (m. sternocleidomastoideus)

M. TERES MINOR – TERES MINOR MUSCLE

SEATED EXTERNAL ROTATION WITH WEIGHTED BALL OR DUMBBELL

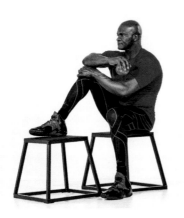

a

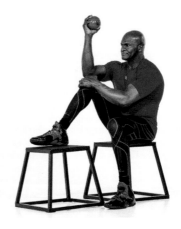

b

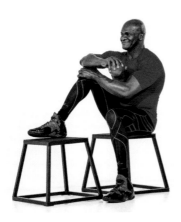

c

Photos 30 a-c

STARTING POSITION

Sit on a stool or on the end of a multipurpose bench. Place one foot on a second stool or on the other end of the bench. The knee is bent. Hold the weighted ball in your hand on the same side and rest the elbow on the bent knee.

EXECUTION

Slowly raise the arm with the weighted ball by externally rotating your shoulder until the forearm is in a vertical position. Now return to the starting position so that the shoulder is stretched slightly. Repeat the exercise and switch arms.

PLEASE NOTE:
Hold the elbow in front of the body at a 90-degree angle at chest or shoulder level during the entire exercise.

PARTICIPATING MUSCLES

PRIMARY
Teres minor muscle (m. teres minor)

SECONDARY
Infraspinatus muscle (m. infraspinatus)

M. TRAPEZIUS, PARS DESCENDENS – UPPER TRAPEZIUS MUSCLE FIBERS
SHRUGS WITH ELASTIC BAND OR CABLE PULLS

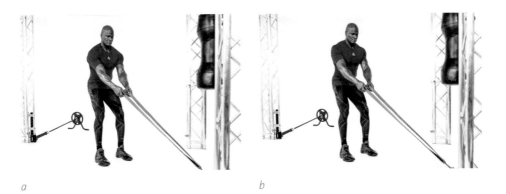

a   b

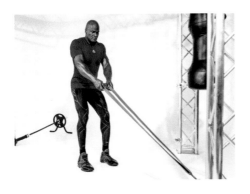

c

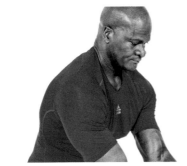
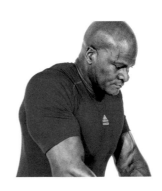

d   e

Photos 31 a-e

STARTING POSITION

Stand facing the band and grip the end with an overhand grip with your hands shoulder-width apart.

EXECUTION

Pull your shoulders as far up and back as possible. Keep your arms extended. Now lower your shoulders and then repeat the exercise.

PLEASE NOTE:

This movement becomes more difficult with a maximum shoulder lift. Depending on an individual's build it can also be enough to just lift the shoulders to a horizontal position.

PARTICIPATING MUSCLES

PRIMARY

Upper trapezius muscle fibers (m. trapezius, pars descendens)

SECONDARY

Middle trapezius muscle fibers (m. trapezius, pars transversa)
Levator scapulae muscle (m. levator scapulae)

M. TRAPEZIUS, PARS DESCENDENS – UPPER TRAPEZIUS MUSCLE FIBERS

SHRUGS WITH WEIGHTED BALLS OR DUMBBELLS

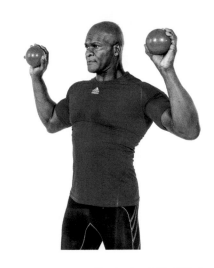

a

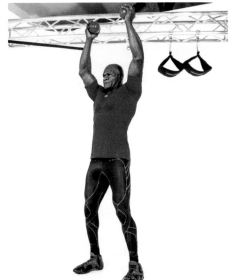

b

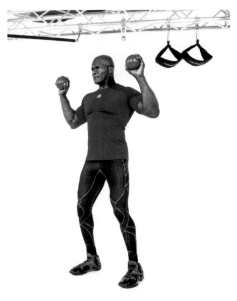

c

Photos 32 a-c

STARTING POSITION

Stand upright. Hold the weights in your hands at head level with your elbows bent. Palms face forward.

EXECUTION

Extend your arms upward and then reach up out of the shoulder joint. Then return to the starting position.

PARTICIPATING MUSCLES

PRIMARY

Upper trapezius muscle fibers (m. trapezius, pars descendens)

SECONDARY

Deltoid muscle, middle head (m. deltoideus, pars acromialis)
Middle trapezius muscle fibers (m. trapezius, pars transversa)

M. TRAPEZIUS, PARS TRANSVERSA – MIDDLE TRAPEZIUS MUSCLE FIBERS
ROWING – SUPINE ROW WITH SLING TRAINER

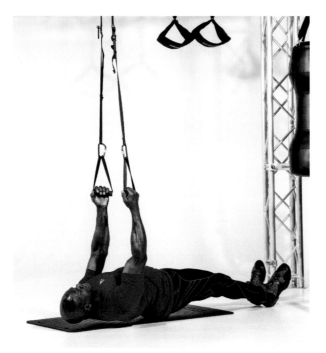

a

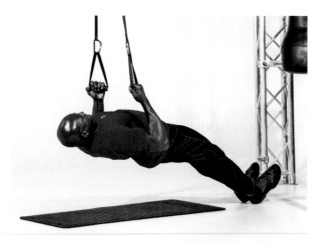

b

Photos 33 a-b

STARTING POSITION

Lie on your back below the sling trainer. Grip the hand loops, rising up so your trunk no longer touches the ground.

EXECUTION

Pull your body up toward the ceiling by bending the elbows. As you move, the body forms a straight line. Now lower it back down until your arms are extended and the shoulders stretched; then repeat the exercise.

PLEASE NOTE:

The hand loops should hang high enough so the body is just above the ground when arms are fully extended. Hand loops can be set higher to lower the resistance and the degree of difficulty, or the exercise can be performed in a seated position. To increase the degree of difficulty, rest your heels on a raised surface. This exercise is usually done without added resistance, but an additional weight can be placed on the abdomen or pelvis.

PARTICIPATING MUSCLES

PRIMARY

Middle trapezius muscle fibers (m. trapezius, pars transversa)
Lower trapezius muscle fibers (m. trapezius, pars ascendens)
Latissimus dorsi muscle (m. latissimus dorsi)

SECONDARY

Teres major muscle (m. teres major)
Deltoid muscle, posterior head (m. deltoideus, pars spinalis)
Infraspinatus muscle (m. infraspinatus)
Teres minor muscle (m. teres minor)
Brachialis muscle (m. brachialis)
Brachioradialis muscle (m. brachioradialis)

M. TRAPEZIUS, PARS TRANSVERSA – MIDDLE TRAPEZIUS MUSCLE FIBERS

BENT-OVER ROW WITH BARBELL

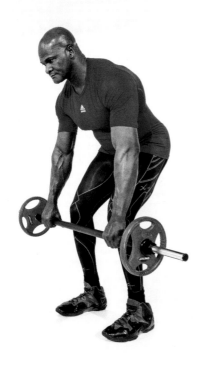 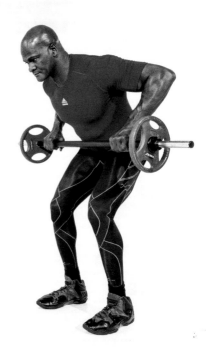

a   b

Photos 34 a-b

STARTING POSITION

Bend toward the barbell with your knees slightly bent and your back straight. Grip the barbell with a wide overhand grip.

EXECUTION

Pull the barbell to your abdomen. Now return to the starting position so the arms are completely extended and shoulders stretched. Repeat the exercise.

PLEASE NOTE:

For a more precise execution, the trunk can be in a nearly horizontal position. Knees are bent so the lower back can remain straight. If the lower back rounds because the muscles in the back of the thighs are tight, bend your knees more or don't drop your upper body as low. Both options can affect the participation of the latissimus dorsi muscles because these positions inevitably require more transverse shoulder extension and less range of motion. If the lower back rounds due to poor physical condition, lift the resting weight to a standing position and then lower the trunk into a horizontal position. Here the knees are bent and the back is straight. A shoulder-width grip or an underhand grip can increase participation of the latissimus dorsi because emphasis is placed on shoulder extension. A wide overhand grip facilitates participation of the entire back musculature and places slight emphasis on the posterior deltoid muscle, infraspinatus muscle, and teres minor muscle.

PARTICIPATING MUSCLES

PRIMARY
Middle trapezius muscle fibers (m. trapezius, pars transversa)
Lower trapezius muscle fibers (m. trapezius, pars ascendens)
Latissimus dorsi muscle (m. latissimus dorsi)

SECONDARY
Teres major muscle (m. teres major)
Deltoid muscle, posterior head (m. deltoideus, pars spinalis)
Infraspinatus muscle (m. infraspinatus)
Teres minor muscle (m. teres minor)
Brachialis muscle (m. brachialis)
Brachioradialis muscle (m. brachioradialis)

M. LATISSIMUS DORSI / M. TERES MAJOR – LATISSIUMUS DORSI MUSCLE / TERES MAJOR MUSCLE

PULL-UP

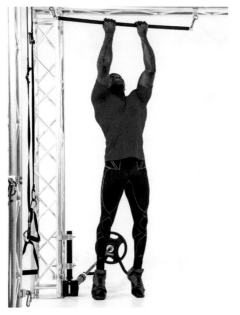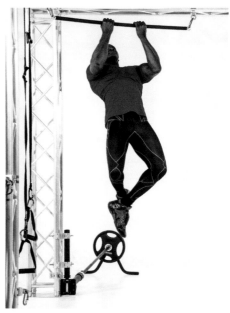

a

b

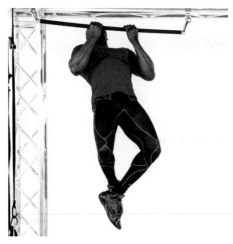

c

Photos 35 a-c

118

STARTING POSITION

Grip the bar with an overhand grip with hands shoulder-width apart.

EXECUTION

Bend the elbows and pull your body up until your chin is level with the bar or slightly higher. Then lower your body so that your arms are fully extended again.

PLEASE NOTE:
The speed should be very controlled during the up and down movement, meaning more slow rather than fast and energetic.

PARTICIPATING MUSCLES

PRIMARY
Latissimus dorsi muscle (m. latissimus dorsi)

SECONDARY
Brachialis muscle (m. brachialis)
Brachioradialis muscle (m. brachioradialis)
Biceps (m. biceps brachii)
Teres major muscle (m. teres major)
Levator scapulae muscle (m. levator scapulae)
Lower trapezius muscle fibers (m. trapezius, pars ascendens)
Rhomboid major muscle (m. rhomboideus major)
Rhomboid minor muscle (m. rhomboideus minor)
Subscapularis muscle (m. subscapularis)
Deltoid muscle, posterior head (m. deltoideus, pars spinalis)

M. LATISSIMUS DORSI / M. TERES MAJOR – LATISSIMUS DORSI MUSCLE / TERES MAJOR MUSCLE

TWO-ARM ROW WITH DUMBBELLS

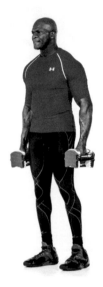

a

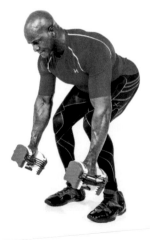

b

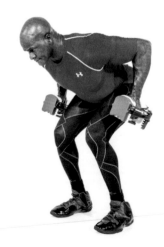

c

Photos 36 a-c

STARTING POSITION

Hold a dumbbell in each hand. Bend your knees and push your posterior back as far as possible. The dumbbells are now just above the floor and slightly to the sides and front of your body. The back remains straight throughout.

EXECUTION

Pull the dumbbells up to your sides at abdomen level. At the same time squeeze your shoulder blades together and bend the elbows (pull back and up). The back remains straight. Return to starting position.

PARTICIPATING MUSCLES

PRIMARY
Latissimus dorsi muscle (m. latissimus dorsi)

SECONDARY
Biceps (m. biceps brachii)
Middle trapezius muscle fibers (m. trapezius, pars transversa)
Rhomboid major muscle (m. rhomboideus major)
Rhomboid minor muscle (m. rhomboideus minor)

M. LATISSIMUS DORSI MUSCLE

PULLDOWNS WITH ELASTIC BAND AND FITNESS BALL

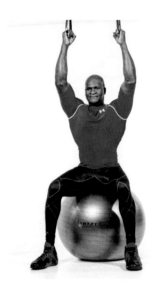

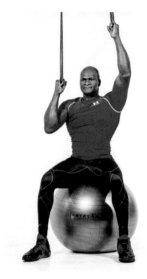

a

b

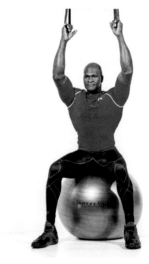

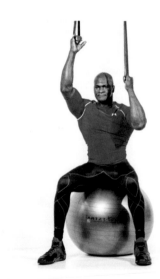

c

d

Photos 37 a-d

STARTING POSITION

Sit on the ball and grip the ends of the band. The entire muscle chain of the lower extremities is taut.

EXECUTION

Alternate pulling one end of the elastic band from above your head down to head level.

PARTICIPATING MUSCLES

PRIMARY
Latissimus dorsi muscle (m. latissimus dorsi)

SECONDARY
Biceps (m. biceps brachii)
Brachioradialis muscle (m. brachioradialis)
Rhomboid major muscle (m. rhomboideus major)
Rhomboid minor muscle (m. rhomboideus minor)
Teres major muscle (m. teres major)
Deltoid muscle, posterior head (m. deltoideus, pars spinalis)
Levator scapulae muscle (m. levator scapulae)
Middle trapezius muscle fibers (m. trapezius, pars transversa)
Lower trapezius muscle fibers (m. trapezius, pars ascendens)
Pectoralis minor muscle (m. pectoralis minor)

M. LATISSIMUS DORSI – LATISSIUMUS DORSI MUSCLE

ONE-ARM ROW WITH KETTLEBELL

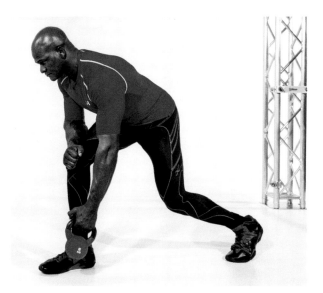

a

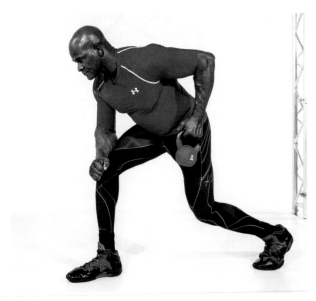

b

Photos 38 a-b

STARTING POSITION

Lunge. Push your posterior as far back as possible and rest your right hand on your right thigh. Your body weight is equally distributed between both feet and the back is straight. Hold the kettlebell in your left hand.

EXECUTION

Lift the kettlebell to your side at abdomen level. At the same time squeeze your shoulder blades together and bend your elbows (pull back and up). The back remains straight throughout. Return to the starting position. Switch sides.

PARTICIPATING MUSCLES

PRIMARY
Latissimus dorsi muscle (m. latissimus dorsi)

SECONDARY
Biceps (m. biceps brachii)
Middle trapezius muscle fibers (m. trapezius, pars transversa)
Rhomboid major muscle (m. rhomboideus major)
Rhomboid minor muscle (m. rhomboideus minor)

M. LATISSIMUS DORSI / M. TRICEPS BRACHII – LATISSIMUS DORSI MUSCLE / TRICEPS

CRAB WALK

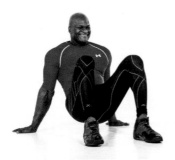

a

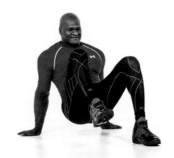

b

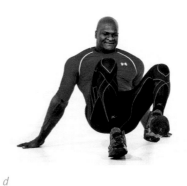

c

d

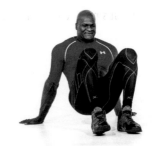

e

f

Photos 39 a-f

STARTING POSITION

Crab walk backward with hand and foot support. Fully extend your arms and bend your knees to 90 degrees. The head is an extension of the spine, and the trunk muscles are engaged.

EXECUTION

You will move sideways in this position. Begin with the inside foot followed by the outside arm and vice versa. Continue this opposing movement pattern.

PARTICIPATING MUSCLES

PRIMARY

Deltoid muscle, posterior head (m. deltoideus, pars spinalis)
Triceps, medial head (m. triceps brachii, caput mediale)
Triceps, long head (m. triceps brachii, caput longum)
Triceps, lateral head (m. triceps brachii, caput laterale)
Latissimus dorsi muscle (m. latissimus dorsi)
Rhomboid major muscle (m. rhomboideus major)
Rhomboid minor muscle (m. rhomboideus minor)
Middle trapezius muscle fibers (m. trapezius, pars transversa)
Lower trapezius muscle fibers (m. trapezius, pars ascendens)
Biceps femoris (m. biceps femoris)
Semitendinosus muscle (m. semitendinosus)
Semimembranosus muscle (m. semimembranosus)

SECONDARY

Multifidus muscle (mm. multifidii)
Longissimus thoracis muscle (m. longissimus thoracis)
Internal obliques (m. obliquus internus abdominis)
External obliques (m. obliquus externus abdominis)

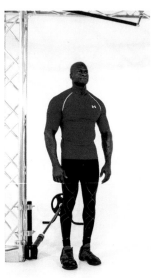
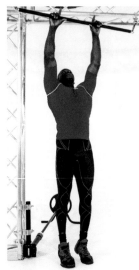
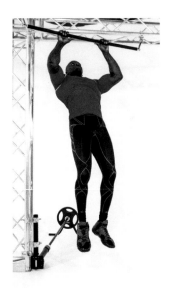

a   *b*   *c*

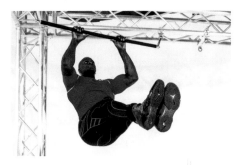

d

Photos 40 a-d

STARTING POSITION

Grip the bar using an overhand grip with hands shoulder-width apart and elbows bent at approximately 90 degrees. Legs are almost fully extended.

EXECUTION

From this position, lift your legs until they are parallel to the floor. Lower your legs and repeat the exercise.

PLEASE NOTE:
The trunk does not move during the entire exercise (no swinging motion).

PARTICIPATING MUSCLES

PRIMARY

Biceps (m. biceps brachii)

Flexor carpi ulnaris muscle (m. flexor carpi ulnaris)

Extensor carpi ulnaris muscle (m. extensor carpi ulnaris)

Extensor digitorum muscle (m. extensor digitorum)

Extensor digiti minimi muscle (m. extensor digiti minimi)

Extensor carpi radialis muscle (m. extensor carpi radialis)

Extensor carpi radialis longus muscle (m. extensor carpi radialis longus)

Brachioradialis muscle (m. brachioradialis)

Flexor carpi radialis muscle (m. flexor carpi radialis)

Palmaris longus muscle (m. palmaris longus)

Flexor digitorum superficialis muscle (m. flexor digitorum superficialis)

Pronator teres muscle (m. pronator teres)

Latissimus dorsi muscle (m. latissimus dorsi)

Iliacus muscle (m. iliacus)

Psoas major muscle (m. psoas major)

SECONDARY

Tensor fasciae latae muscle (m. tensor fasciae latae)

Pectineus muscle (m. pectineus)

Sartorius muscle (m. sartorius)

Long adductor muscle (m. adductor longus)

Short adductor muscle (m. adductor brevis)

Rectus abdominis muscle (m. rectus abdominis)

External oblique muscle (m. obliquus externus abdominis)

Internal oblique muscle (m. obliquus internus abdominis)

M. DELTOIDEUS – DELTOID MUSCLE, MIDDLE HEAD
SHOULDER 90 DEGREES DYNAMIC

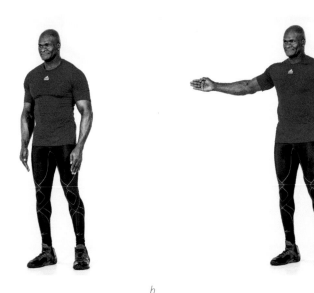

a   b

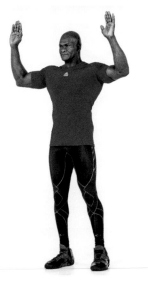 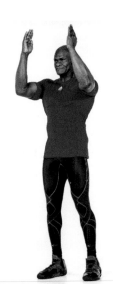

c   d

Photos 41 a-d

STARTING POSITION

Stand with your feet hip-width apart, arms hanging at your sides.

EXECUTION

Raise the arms to the side, up to shoulder level, and bend the elbows approximately 90 degrees. Keeping your arms at this level, bring your elbows together in front of your body. Then move your arms back to the side and repeat the exercise.

PLEASE NOTE:
Elbows remain bent and the neck is relaxed. The head is an extension of the spine, and the eyes look straight ahead. Intensity changes with motion speed.

PARTICIPATING MUSCLES

PRIMARY
Deltoid muscle, middle head (m. deltoideus, pars acromialis)
Deltoid muscle, anterior head (m. deltoideus, pars clavicularis)

SECONDARY
Serratus anterior muscle (m. serratus anterior)
Biceps (m. biceps brachii)
Pectoralis major, clavicular head (m. pectoralis major, pars clavicularis)
Teres major muscle (m. teres major)
Infraspinatus muscle (m. infraspinatus)
Supraspinatus muscle (m. supraspinatus)

M. DELTOIDEUS – DELTOID MUSCLE, MIDDLE HEAD

SHADOW BOXING – UPPER CUT

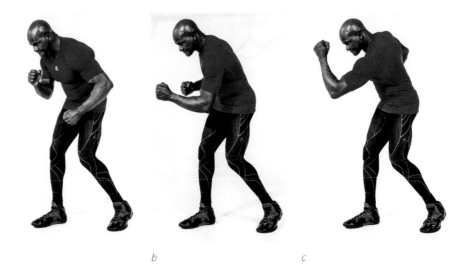

a   b   c

Photos 42 a-c

STARTING POSITION

Get into a slight lunge position with your legs shoulder-width apart. Bend your elbows in front of your body like a boxer in defensive position.

EXECUTION

Punch upward as though you were striking an opponent. With each punch, turn your body and bring your hip forward. Immediately after, repeat the exercise with the other arm. After each punch, return to the starting position.

PLEASE NOTE:

Turn your upper body to increase the power of the punch. Don't forget to breathe during the exercise.

PARTICIPATING MUSCLES

PRIMARY

Deltoid muscle, anterior head (m. deltoideus, pars clavicularis)

Deltoid muscle, middle head (m. deltoideus, pars acromialis)

Deltoid muscle, posterior head (m. deltoideus, pars spinalis)

Pectoralis major, sternal head (m. pectoralis major, pars sternocostalis)

Pectoralis major, abdominal head (m. pectoralis major, pars abdominalis)

Pectoralis major, clavicular head (m. pectoralis major, pars clavicularis)

Teres major muscle (m. teres major)

Teres minor muscle (m. teres minor)

Latissimus dorsi muscle (m. latissimus dorsi)

Infraspinatus muscle (m. infraspinatus)

Pronator teres muscle (m. pronator teres)

Brachialis muscle (m. brachialis)

Brachioradialis muscle (m. brachioradialis)

Rhomboid major muscle (m. rhomboideus major)

Rhomboid minor muscle (m. rhomboideus minor)

SECONDARY

External oblique muscle (m. obliquus externus abdominis)

Internal oblique muscle (m. obliquus internus abdominis)

Rectus abdominis muscle (m. rectus abdominis)

M. DELTOIDEUS – DELTOID MUSCLE, MIDDLE HEAD

SCARECROW WITH DUMBBELLS ON LARGE FITNESS BALL

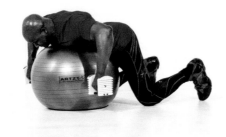

a

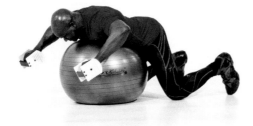

b

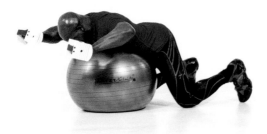

c

Photos 43 a-c

STARTING POSITION

Begin with your abdomen on the ball. Hold one dumbbell in each hand with an overhand grip. Forearms are in a vertical position with hands to the side of the fitness ball.

EXECUTION

Lift the dumbbells forward and up until your forearms are parallel to the floor, hands toward the ceiling. Briefly hold and then return to the starting position.

PARTICIPATING MUSCLES

PRIMARY

Deltoid muscle, middle head (m. deltoideus, pars acromialis)
Deltoid muscle, middle head (m. deltoideus, pars acromialis)

SECONDARY

Middle trapezius muscle fibers (m. trapezius, pars transversa)
Upper trapezius muscle fibers (m. trapezius, pars descendens)

M. DELTOIDEUS – DELTOID MUSCLE, ANTERIOR HEAD

TWISTED PRESS WITH ELASTIC BAND RESISTANCE

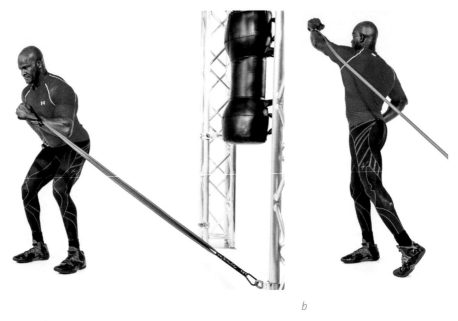

a   b

Photos 44 a-b

STARTING POSITION

Stand next to an elastic band mounted low or at medium height. Hold the grip in front of the shoulder with the hand closest to the band. The elbow is at the side of the body. Prop the other hand against the hip. Plant your feet approximately shoulder-width apart and get into a slight squat.

EXECUTION

Turn the body away from the attachment point, extend the legs, and push the handle diagonally upward toward the other side of the body. Now slowly return to the starting position and repeat the exercise.

PLEASE NOTE:
Internal rotation of the hip is considerably greater than the spinal rotation.

PARTICIPATING MUSCLES

PRIMARY

Deltoid muscle, anterior head (m. deltoideus, pars clavicularis)
Triceps muscle, lateral head (m. triceps brachii, caput laterale)
Triceps muscle, long head (m. triceps brachii, caput longum)
Triceps muscle, medial head (m. triceps brachii, caput mediale)

SECONDARY

Deltoid muscle, middle head (m. deltoideus, pars acromialis)
Triceps muscle, lateral head (m. triceps brachii, caput laterale)
Triceps muscle, long head (m. triceps brachii, caput longum)
Triceps muscle, medial head (m. triceps brachii, caput mediale)
Middle trapezius muscle fibers (m. trapezius, pars transversa)
Lower trapezius muscle fibers (m. trapezius, pars ascendens)
Serratus anterior muscle (m. serratus anterior)
Gluteus maximus muscle (m. gluteus maximus)
Adductor magnus muscle (m. adductor magnus)
Rectus femoris muscle (m. rectus femoris)
Vastus lateralis muscle (m. vastus lateralis)
Soleus muscle (m. soleus)
External oblique muscle (m. obliquus externus abdominis)
Internal oblique muscle (m. obliquus internus abdominis)
Psoas major muscle (m. psoas major)
Iliocostalis muscle (m. iliocostalis)
Tensor fasciae latae muscle (m. flexor fasciae latae)
Gluteus medius muscle (m. gluteus medius)
Supraspinatus muscle (m. supraspinatus)
Vastus intermedius muscle (m. vastus intermedius)
Quadratus lumborum muscle (m. quadratus lumborum)

M. DELTOIDEUS – DELTOID MUSCLE, ANTERIOR HEAD

JERK, SPLIT - CLEAN AND JERK WITH BARBELL

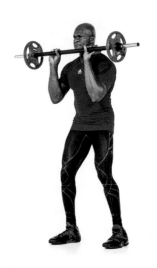
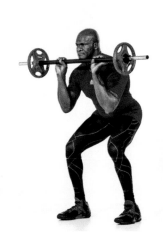
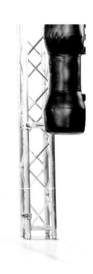

a   b

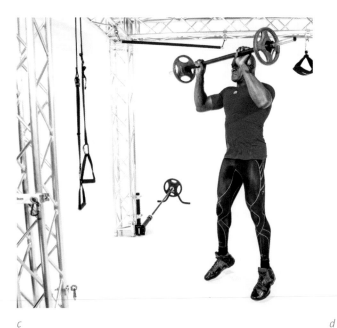
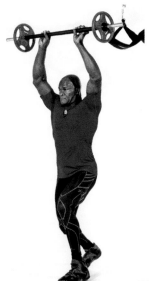

c   d

Photos 45 a-d

STARTING POSITION

Begin in a standing position with feet shoulder-width apart.

EXECUTION

Slightly bend your knees to prepare for a jump. Then jump up and simultaneously thrust the barbell up overhead and land in a lunge position. Slowly return to the starting position.

PARTICIPATING MUSCLES

PRIMARY
Deltoid muscle, anterior head (m. deltoideus, pars clavicularis)

SECONDARY
Gastrocnemius muscle, medial head (m. gastrocnemius, caput mediale)

Gastrocnemius muscle, lateral head (m. gastrocnemius, caput laterale)

Gluteus medius muscle (m. gluteus medius)

Gluteus maximus muscle (m. gluteus maximus)

Rectus femoris muscle m. rectus femoris)

Vastus medialis muscle (m. vastus medialis)

Vastus lateralis muscle (m. vastus lateralis)

Vastus intermedius muscle (m. vastus intermedius)

Soleus muscle (m. soleus)

M. DELTOIDEUS – DELTOID MUSCLE, MIDDLE HEAD
LATERAL RAISE WITH RESISTANCE (GYM STICK/TUBE OR CABLE)

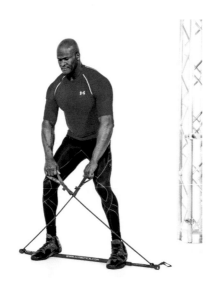

a

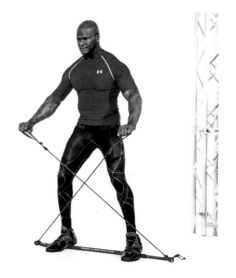

b

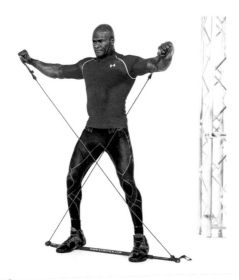

c

Photos 46 a-c

STARTING POSITION

Stand upright between two pulls. Hold the left grip in the right hand and the right grip in the left hand.

EXECUTION

Raise your arms to shoulder level, keeping your elbows slightly bent. Now slowly lower the arms and repeat the exercise.

PLEASE NOTE:
The elbows remain slightly bent during the entire exercise. The grips are raised using shoulder abduction, not external rotation.

PARTICIPATING MUSCLES

PRIMARY
Deltoid muscle, middle head (m. deltoideus, pars acromialis)

SECONDARY
Deltoid muscle, anterior head (m. deltoideus, pars clavicularis)
Middle trapezius muscle fibers (m. trapezius, pars transversa)
Lower trapezius muscle fibers (m. trapezius, pars ascendens)
Serratus anterior muscle (m. serratus anterior)
Supraspinatus muscle (m. supraspinatus)

CHEST AND SHOULDER

M. PECTORALIS/M. DELTOIDEUS – PECTORALIS MAJOR MUSCLE/DELTOID MUSCLE, ANTERIOR HEAD

KETTLEBELL FLOOR PRESS – EXTENDED RANGE

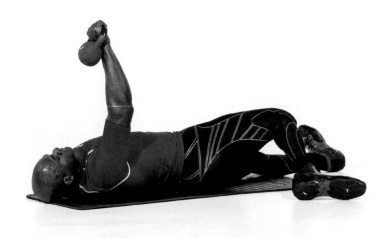

a

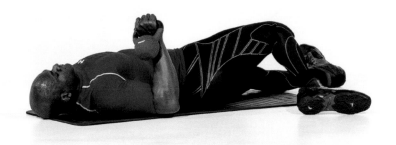

b

Photos 47 a-b

STARTING POSITION

Lie down on your side. Turn your upper body so your upper back rests on the floor. The hip does not move. Press the weight straight up until the arm is completely extended.

EXECUTION

Lower the weight toward the chest, rotating the wrist toward the body's midline. Then return to the starting position.

PARTICIPATING MUSCLES

PRIMARY

Pectoralis major muscle, sternal head (m. pectoralis major, pars sternocostalis)

SECONDARY

Deltoid muscle, anterior head (m. deltoideus, pars clavicularis)
Triceps muscle, long head (m. triceps brachii, caput longum)
Triceps muscle, lateral head (m. triceps brachii, caput laterale)

M. PECTORALIS/M. DELTOIDEUS – PECTORALIS MAJOR MUSCLE/DELTOID MUSCLE, POSTERIOR HEAD

PULLOVER WITH ELBOWS BENT ON LARGE FITNESS BALL WITH DUMBBELLS OR WEIGHTED BALL

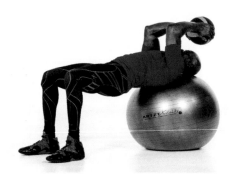

a

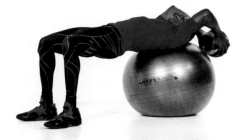

b

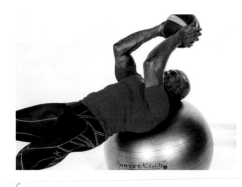

c

d

Photos 48 a-d

STARTING POSITION

Begin with your back on the ball. Hold the weighted ball overhead with both hands and elbows bent. Forearms are parallel to the floor and at a right angle to the upper arms.

EXECUTION

Slowly lower the weighted ball behind your head until your upper arms are parallel to the floor and forearms perpendicular. As you do so, keep your elbows bent. Now return to the starting position.

PARTICIPATING MUSCLES

PRIMARY

Pectoralis major muscle, sternal head (m. pectoralis major, pars sternocostalis)

SECONDARY

Triceps muscle, long head (m. triceps brachii, caput longum)
Triceps muscle, lateral head (m. triceps brachii, caput laterale)
Deltoid muscle, posterior head (m. deltoideus, pars spinalis)
Latissimus dorsi muscle (m. latissius dorsi)
Pectoralis minor muscle (m. pectoralis minor)
Brachialis muscle (m. brachialis)
Rhomboid major muscle (m. rhomboideus major)
Rhomboid minor muscle (m. rhomboideus minor)
Teres major muscle (m. teres major)
Teres minor muscle (m. teres minor)
Levator scapulae muscle (m. levator scapulae)

M. PECTORALIS/M. DELTOIDEUS – PECTORALIS MAJOR MUSCLE/DELTOID MUSCLE, POSTERIOR HEAD

SQUAT HOLD

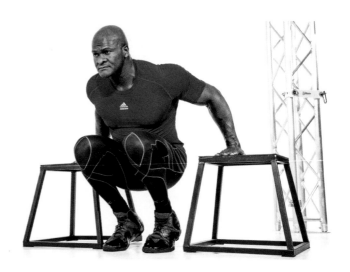

a

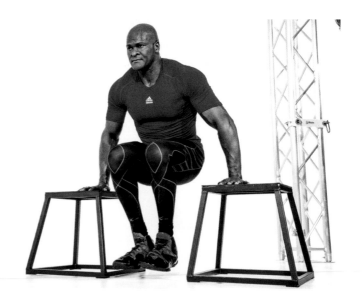

b

Photos 49 a-b

STARTING POSITION

Stand between two raised surfaces that are of equal height and able to support your body weight.

EXECUTION

Squat down and place your hands on the surfaces. Extend your arms. Now lift your knees until your thighs and calves are at right angles to each other. Hold this position as long as you can. Lower your legs and repeat the exercise.

PLEASE NOTE:
During this exercise the head is an extension of the spine, and the trunk muscles are engaged. Shoulders pull back and toes point forward.

PARTICIPATING MUSCLES

PRIMARY
Deltoid muscle, middle head (m. deltoideus, pars acromialis)
Pectoralis major, clavicular head (m. pectoralis major, pars clavicularis)
Pectoralis major muscle, sternal head (m. pectoralis major, pars sternocostalis)
Middle trapezius muscle fibers (m. trapezius, pars transversa)
Biceps muscle (m. biceps brachii)

SECONDARY
Infraspinatus muscle (m. infraspinatus)
Supraspinatus muscle (m. supraspinatus)

M. PECTORALIS/M. DELTOIDEUS – PECTORALIS MAJOR MUSCLE/DELTOID MUSCLE

HAND STEP-UPS ON UNSTABLE SURFACES

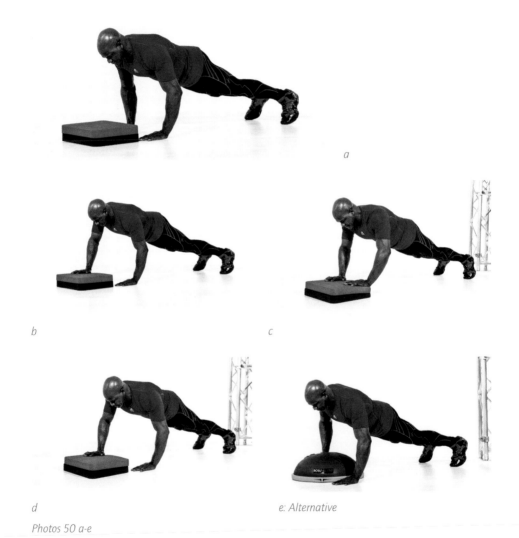

a

b

c

d

e: Alternative

Photos 50 a-e

STARTING POSITION

You begin in push-up position behind an unstable surface. Hands are shoulder-width apart and feet are hip-width apart. The head is an extension of the spine, and the body forms a straight line.

EXECUTION

Raise one arm and set that hand on the unstable surface. The other hand immediately follows. Then both hands return to the starting position. Continue to repeat this exercise.

PLEASE NOTE:
Be careful not to push the chin forward, and don't let the hips sag. Work at a constant pace, and keep the trunk muscles engaged while moving. To increase the degree of difficulty, move your hands farther apart or change the pace. The starting position of the hands can be in front of or next to the unstable surface.

PARTICIPATING MUSCLES

PRIMARY
Deltoid muscle, middle head (m. deltoideus, pars acromialis)
Deltoid muscle, anterior head (m. deltoideus, pars clavicularis)
Deltoid muscle, posterior head (m. deltoideus, pars spinalis)
Pectoralis major, sternal head (m. pectoralis major, pars sternocostalis)
Pectoralis major, clavicular head (m. pectoralis major, pars clavicularis)

SECONDARY
Rhomboid major muscle (m. rhomboideus major)
Rhomboid minor muscle (m. rhomboideus minor)
Middle trapezius muscle fibers (m. trapezius, pars transversa)

M. PECTORALIS/M. DELTOIDEUS – PECTORALIS MAJOR MUSCLE/DELTOID MUSCLE, ANTERIOR HEAD

ASSISTED DIPS WITH ELASTIC BANDS

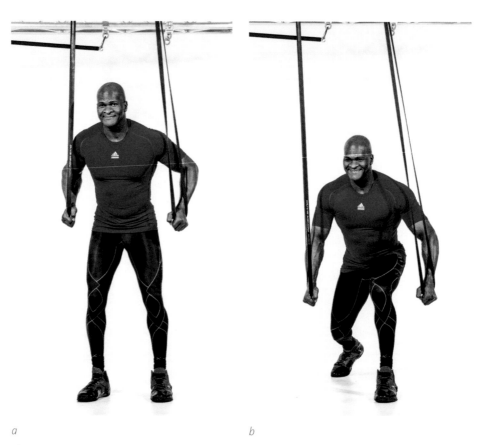

a   b

Photos 51 a-b

STARTING POSITION

Grip the bands with palms down at hip level, stabilizing your trunk and opening your feet to shoulder-width to prepare the entire muscle chain required for the dip.

EXECUTION

Prepare by slightly bending the elbows (elbows move slightly to the outside). As soon as you feel a slight stretch in the chest and shoulder area, press the bands toward the floor until your arms are fully extended, and at the same time perform a back lunge. Repeat the exercise while lunging with the other leg.

PLEASE NOTE:

This exercise is a functional dynamic dip and, therefore, requires a standing starting position and a back lunge. For beginners, there are machines that help provide a similar exercise execution in a kneeling position (assisted).

PARTICIPATING MUSCLES

PRIMARY

Pectoralis major, sternal head (m. pectoralis major, pars sternocostalis)
Pectoralis major, abdominal head (m. pectoralis major, pars abdominalis)

SECONDARY

Deltoid muscle, anterior head (m. deltoideus, pars clavicularis)
Triceps muscle, lateral head (m. triceps brachii, caput laterale)
Triceps muscle, long head (m. triceps brachii, caput longum)
Triceps muscle, lower inside head (m. triceps brachii, caput mediale)
Levator scapulae muscle (m. levator scapulae)
Latissimus dorsi muscle (m. latissimus dorsi)
Teres major muscle (m. teres major)
Pectoralis minor (m. pectoralis minor)

M. PECTORALIS / M. DELTOIDEUS – PECTORALIS MAJOR MUSCLE / DELTOID MUSCLE, ANTERIOR HEAD

T PUSH-UP

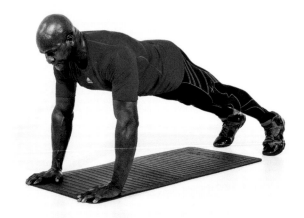

a

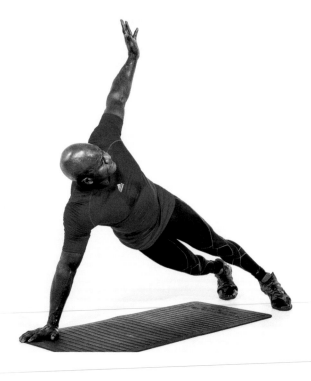

b

Photos 52 a-b

STARTING POSITION

Get into push-up position with arms extended.

EXECUTION

While in push-up position, rotate your trunk, lift one hand off the floor and extend that arm toward the ceiling. Hold the body in a straight line (toes remain planted). Now repeat the exercise on the other side.

PARTICIPATING MUSCLES

PRIMARY

Pectoralis major, clavicular head (m. pectoralis major, pars clavicularis)
Pectoralis major, sternal head (m. pectoralis major, pars sternocostalis)

SECONDARY

External oblique muscle (m. obliquus externus abdominis)
Internal oblique muscle (m. obliquus internus abdominis)
Triceps muscle, long head (m. triceps brachii, caput longum)
Triceps muscle, lateral head (m. triceps brachii, caput laterale)
Deltoid muscle, anterior head (m. deltoideus, pars clavicularis)

ABDOMEN

M. RECTUS ABDOMINIS – RECTUS ABDOMINIS MUSCLE

PLANK – ALTERNATING ARM AND LEG EXTENSIONS

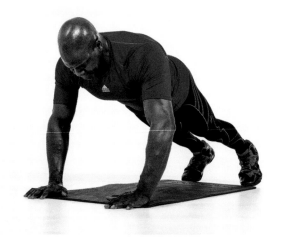

a

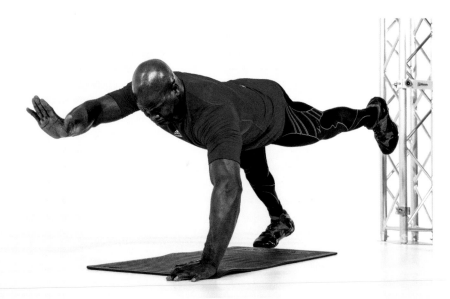

b

Photos 53 a-b

STARTING POSITION

Get into push-up position on your toes with your hands shoulder-width apart. The head is an extension of the spine, and the back is straight.

EXECUTION

Extend one arm forward while at the same time extending the opposite leg back until both arm and leg are fully extended. Now bring the arm and opposite leg together. Then repeat the exercise and switch sides.

PLEASE NOTE:

During the movement, the head is an extension of the spine, and the abdominal muscles are engaged. Extend arms and legs until they are parallel to the floor. Beginners can do this exercise on their knees.

PARTICIPATING MUSCLES

PRIMARY

Rectus abdominis muscle (m. rectus abdominis)

SECONDARY

External oblique muscle (m. obliquus externus abdominis)
Internal oblique muscle (m. obliquus internus abdominis)
Iliacus muscle (m. iliacus)
Psoas major muscle (m. psoas major)
Sartorius muscle (m. Sartorius)
Pectoralis major (m. pectoralis major)
Serratus anterior muscle (m. serratus anterior)
Pectoralis major, sternal head (m. pectoralis major, pars sternocostalis)
Vastus lateralis muscle (m. vastus lateralis)
Vastus intermedius muscle (m. vastus intermedius)
Vastus medialis muscle (m. vastus medialis)

M. RECTUS ABDOMINIS – RECTUS ABDOMINIS MUSCLE

HIP RAISE

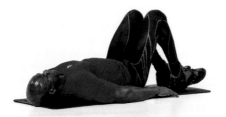

a

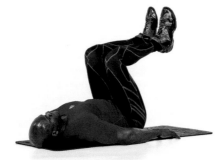

b

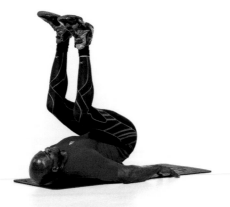

c

Photos 54 a-c

STARTING POSITION

Lie on your back. Both feet are planted flat on the floor, and arms are resting alongside the body.

EXECUTION

Lift your legs and hips off the floor so your knees move slightly toward your head (forward and up) and the lower back no longer touches the floor. The arms only help to stabilize and should support raising the hips as little as possible.

PARTICIPATING MUSCLES

PRIMARY
Rectus abdominis muscle (m. rectus abdominis)

SECONDARY
External oblique muscle (m. obliquus externus abdominis)
Internal oblique muscle (m. obliquus internus abdominis)
Multifidus muscle (mm. multifidii)
Quadratus lumborum muscle (m. quadratus lumborum)
Longissimus thoracis muscle (m. longissimus thoracis)
Latissimus dorsi muscle (m. latissimus dorsi)

M. RECTUS ABDOMINIS – RECTUS ABDOMINIS MUSCLE

FOREARM PLANK JACKS

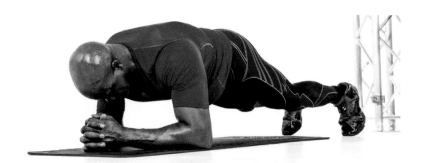

a

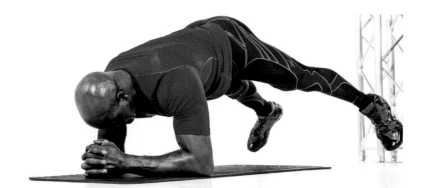

b

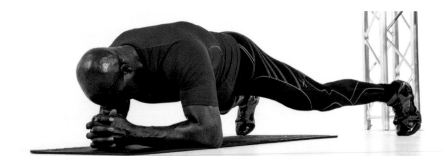

c

Photos 55 a-c

STARTING POSITION

On your abdomen, raise your body so only your forearms and toes touch the floor. Keep your back straight.

EXECUTION

For more stability, keep your hands close together. Your body forms a straight line. Now jump your legs more than shoulder-width apart. Briefly stabilize your position and then jump back into the starting position. Repeat the exercise.

PARTICIPATING MUSCLES

PRIMARY

Rectus abdominis muscle (m. rectus abdominis)
Transverse abdominal muscle (m. transversus abdominis)

SECONDARY

External oblique muscle (m. obliquus externus abdominis)
Internal oblique muscle (m. obliquus internus abdominis)
Multifidus muscle (mm. multifidii)
Quadratus lumborum muscle (m. quadratus lumborum)
Longissimus thoracis muscle (m. longissimus thoracis)
Iliocostalis muscle (m. iliocostalis)
Latissimus dorsi muscle (m. latissimus dorsi)

M. RECTUS ABDOMINIS – RECTUS ABDOMINIS MUSCLE

WINDMILL WITH A KETTLEBELL

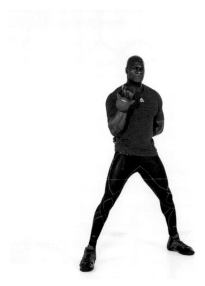

a

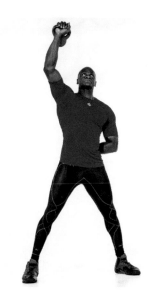

b

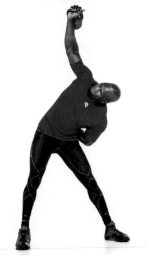

c

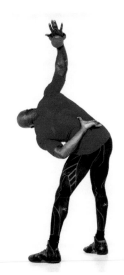

d

Photos 56 a-d

STARTING POSITION

Stand with feet more than shoulder-width apart. Begin by lifting the kettlebell to shoulder level with one arm, and then push it up overhead.

EXECUTION

Firmly grip the kettlebell with your hand and slowly bend forward. At the same time, track the kettlebell with your eyes to create a slight rotation of the trunk. The arm remains extended.

PARTICIPATING MUSCLES

PRIMARY
Rectus abdominis muscle (m. rectus abdominis)
External oblique muscle (m. obliquus externus abdominis)
Internal oblique muscle (m. obliquus internus abdominis)

SECONDARY
Gluteus medius muscle (m. gluteus medius)
Gluteus maximus muscle (m. gluteus maximus)
Biceps femoris muscle (m. biceps femoris)

M. RECTUS ABDOMINIS – RECTUS ABDOMINIS MUSCLE

OVERHEAD CHOP WITH MEDICINE BALL

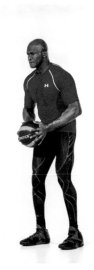

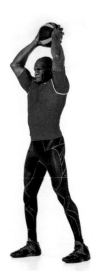

a

b

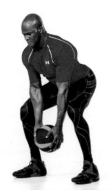

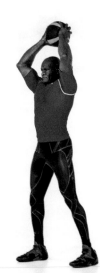

c

d

Photos 57 a-d

162

STARTING POSITION

Stand tall with your feet slightly more than shoulder-width apart. Hold the medicine ball overhead with your elbows slightly bent.

EXECUTION

Bend your knees and lower the medicine ball between your legs. Now return to the starting position.

PARTICIPATING MUSCLES

PRIMARY

Rectus abdominis muscle (m. rectus abdominis)
External oblique muscle (m. obliquus externus abdominis)
Internal oblique muscle (m. obliquus internus abdominis)
Deltoid muscle, anterior head (m. deltoideus, pars clavicularis)

SECONDARY

Vastus lateralis muscle (m. vastus lateralis)
Vastus intermedius muscle (m. vastus intermedius)
Vastus medialis muscle (m. vastus medialis)
Rectus femoris muscle (m. rectus femoris)

M. TRANSVERSUS ABDOMINIS – TRANSVERSE ABDOMINAL MUSCLE

LUMBERJACK

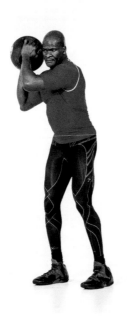

a

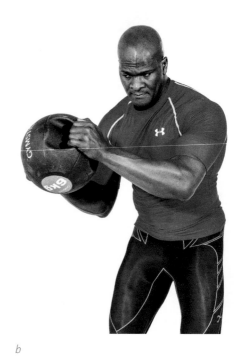

b

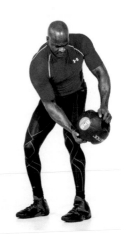

c

Photos 58 a-c

STARTING POSITION

Stand tall with your feet shoulder-width apart. Hold the medicine ball next to your right shoulder. The opposite arm is in front of the upper body. Turn your upper body toward the ball.

EXECUTION

From the starting position, move the medicine ball down diagonally in front of the body to the outside of your left knee. The right knee must bend slightly so you are able to reach this low position. Now return to the starting position, and repeat the exercise on the other side.

PARTICIPATING MUSCLES

PRIMARY
Rectus abdominis muscle (m. rectus abdominis)
External oblique muscle (m. obliquus externus abdominis)
Internal oblique muscle (m. obliquus internus abdominis)

SECONDARY
Transverse abdominal muscle (m. transversus abdominis)

M. TRANSVERSUS ABDOMINIS – TRANSVERSE ABDOMINAL MUSCLE

PLANK – LEG LIFTS WITH SLING TRAINER

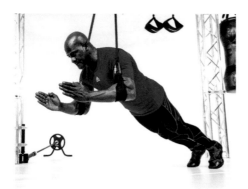

a

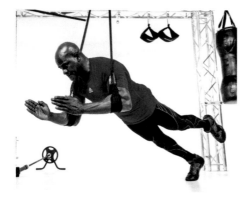

b

Photos 59 a-b

STARTING POSITION

Place your forearms into the sling trainer hand loops and prop yourself on your forearms and toes. Forearms are shoulder-width apart, and feet are hip-width apart. The head is an extension of the spine, and the body forms a straight line.

EXECUTION

Stay in this position and lift one leg. The leg is fully extended, and the hip is straight and parallel to the floor. Now return to the starting position and repeat the exercise with the other leg.

PLEASE NOTE:

Do not tuck the chin to the chest, and don't let your hips sag. The trunk muscles are engaged during the hold. Intensity changes with motion speed.

PARTICIPATING MUSCLES

PRIMARY

External oblique muscle (m. obliquus externus abdominis)
Internal oblique muscle (m. obliquus internus abdominis)

SECONDARY

Gluteus medius muscle (m. gluteus medius)
Gluteus minimus muscle (m. gluteus minimus)
Tensor fasciae latae muscle (m. tensor fasciae latae)
Quadratus lumborum muscle (m. quadratus lumborum)
Psoas major muscle (m. psoas major)
Pectinaeus muscle (m. pectinaeus)
Gracilis muscle (m. gracilis)
Gluteus maximus muscle (m. gluteus maximus)
Latissimus dorsi muscle (m. latissimus dorsi)
Pectoralis minor muscle (m. pectoralis minor)
Pectoralis major muscle, sternal head (m. pectoralis major, pars sternocostalis)
Levator scapulae muscle (m. levator scapulae)
Short adductor muscle (m. adductor brevis)
Long adductor muscle (m. adductor longus)
Adductor magnus muscle (m. adductor magnus)

GLUTEALS

M. GLUTEUS MAXIMUS – GLUTEUS MAXIMUS MUSCLE

HIP EXTENSION WITH ELASTIC BAND

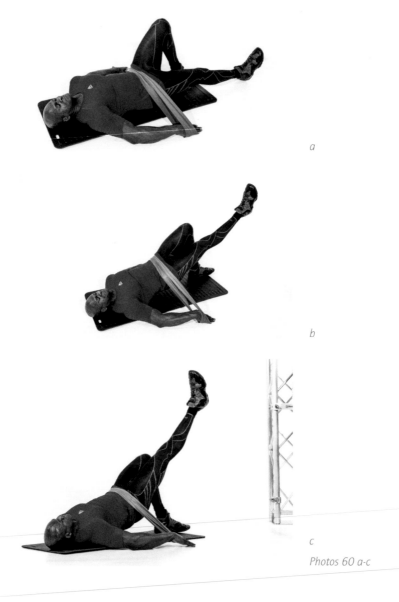

a

b

c

Photos 60 a-c

STARTING POSITION

Lie on your back on the floor or on a mat. Extend one leg and bend the other knee, planting that foot flat on the floor or mat. Arms are on the floor alongside the body, maintaining tension on the band.

EXECUTION

Lift your body against the resistance of the band by straightening the hip on the same side as the bent knee. As you do so, keep the extended leg and hip straight. Now lower your body, continuing to keep the extended leg and hip straight. Repeat the exercise and then switch legs.

PARTICIPATING MUSCLES

PRIMARY
Gluteus maximus (m. gluteus maximus)

M. GLUTEUS MAXIMUS – GLUTEUS MAXIMUS MUSCLE

UPWARD JUMP

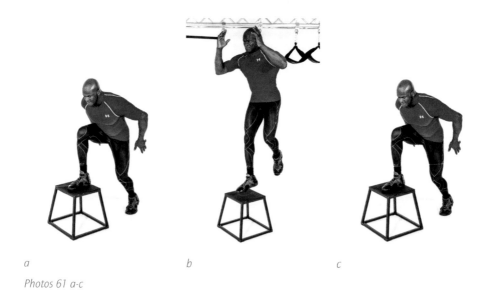

a   b   c

Photos 61 a-c

STARTING POSITION

Stand upright with legs hip-width apart and arms at your sides.

EXECUTION

Place one foot on a raised surface. Quickly bend the knee and hip and immediately jump up as a high as you can. Stay in a lunge position. Land softly and return to the upright starting position. Now repeat the exercise. The forward knee should not jut out over the toes.

PLEASE NOTE:

You will gather additional momentum if you swing your arms in rhythm with the movement. Lift your chest and engage your trunk muscles. To increase the degree of difficulty, you can decrease the amount of time between jumps. Make sure the landing is soft (quiet) and the takeoff motion is impulsive.

PARTICIPATING MUSCLES

PRIMARY

Gluteus maximus (m. gluteus maximus)

Semitendinosus muscle (m. semitendinosus)

Semimembranosus muscle (m. semimembranosus)

Biceps femoris muscle (m. biceps femoris)

Adductor magnus muscle (m. adductor magnus)

Rectus femoris muscle (m. rectus femoris)

Vastus lateralis muscle (m. vastus lateralis)

Vastus medialis muscle (m. vastus medialis)

Vastus intermedius muscle (m. vastus intermedius)

Gastrocnemius muscle, medial head (m. gastrocnemius, caput mediale)

Gastrocnemius muscle, lateral head (m. gastrocnemius, caput laterale)

Soleus muscle (m. soleus)

Achilles tendon

Tibialis anterior muscle (m. tibialis anterior)

Extensor digitorum longus muscle (m. extensor digitorum longus)

SECONDARY

Deltoid muscle, middle head (m. deltoideus, pars acromialis)

Deltoid muscle, anterior head (m. deltoideus, pars clavicularis)

Supraspinatus muscle (m. supraspinatus)

Pectoralis major muscle, clavicular head (m. pectoralis major, pars clavicularis)

Biceps brachii muscle (m. biceps brachii)

Trapezius muscle, lower fibers (m. trapezius, pars ascendens)

Trapezius muscle, middle fibers (m. trapezius, pars transversa)

Serratus anterior muscle (m. serratus anterior)

Rectus abdominis muscle (m. recuts abdominis)

GLUTEALS AND LEGS

M. GLUTEUS/M. PIRIFORMIS – GLUTEAL MUSCLE/PIRIFORMIS MUSCLE

STANDING HIP ABDUCTION WITH ELASTIC RESISTANCE

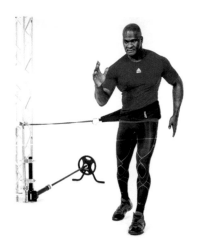
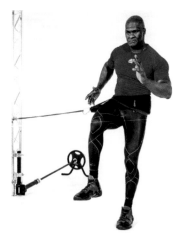

a *b*

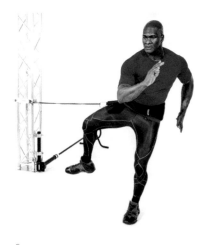
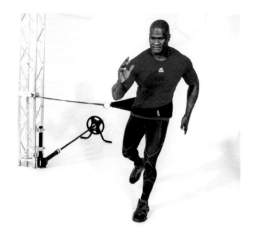

c *d*

Photos 62 a-d

STARTING POSITION

Stand upright with legs hip-width apart. Elbows are bent and raised to support the motion. Lift one leg at a right angle so the thigh is parallel to the floor.

EXECUTION

Externally rotate the knee away from the body as far as you can (abduction). Now return to the starting position (adduction) and repeat the exercise.

PLEASE NOTE:
During the exercise the head is an extension of the spine, and the trunk muscles are engaged. The thigh remains parallel to the floor.

PARTICIPATING MUSCLES

PRIMARY
Gluteus medius (m. gluteus medius)
Gluteus minimus (m. gluteus minimus)
Tensor fasciae latae muscle (m. tensor fasciae latae)

SECONDARY
Sartorius muscle (m. sartorius)
Piriform muscle (m. piriformis)

M. GLUTEUS/ M. PIRIFORMIS – GLUTEAL MUSCLE/PIRIFORMIS MUSCLE

SHUFFLE WITH ELASTIC RESISTANCE

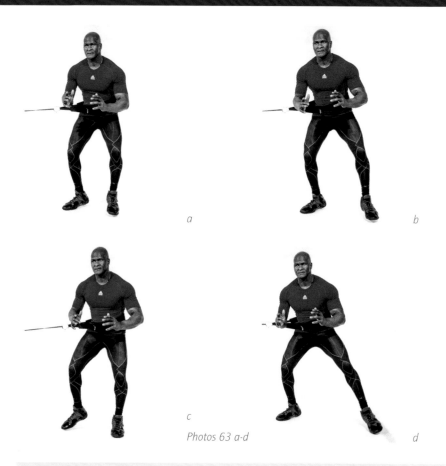

a

b

c

Photos 63 a-d

d

STARTING POSITION

Stand upright with legs hip-width apart. Arms are held loosely at hip level.

EXECUTION

Get into a slight squat. Hips, knees, and ankle joints are slightly flexed. Now move your feet sideways, barely lifting them off the floor. Make sure your feet do not touch and you remain in a slight squat. Repeat the exercise by reversing direction.

PLEASE NOTE:
During the exercise, look straight ahead, and keep your back straight and your trunk muscles engaged. Intensity changes with motion speed.

PARTICIPATING MUSCLES

PRIMARY

Long adductor muscle (m. adductor longus)

Short adductor muscle (m. adductor brevis

Adductor magnus muscle (m. adductor magnus)

Vastus lateralis muscle (m. vastus lateralis)

Vastus medialis muscle (m. vastus medialis)

Vastus intermedius muscle (m. vastus intermedius)

Rectus femoris muscle (m. rectus femoris)

Piriformis muscle (m. piriformis)

Gastrocnemius muscle, medial head (m. gastrocnemius, caput mediale)

Gastrocnemius muscle, lateral head (m. gastrocnemius, caput laterale)

Semitendinosus muscle (m. semitendinosus)

Soleus muscle (m. soleus)

Gluteus maximus (m. gluteus maximus)

Tensor fasciae latae muscle (m. tensor fasciae latae)

Sartorius muscle (m. sartorius)

Gracilis muscle (m. gracilis)

Fibularis longus muscle (m. fibularis longus)

Achilles tendon

SECONDARY

Gluteus medius (m. gluteus medius)

Gluteus minimus (m. gluteus minimus)

External oblique muscle (m. obliquus externus abdominis)

Internal oblique muscle (m. obliquus internus abdominis)

M. GLUTEUS / M. PIRIFORMIS – GLUTEAL MUSCLE / PIRIFORMIS MUSCLE

SIDE TWIST HIP STRETCH

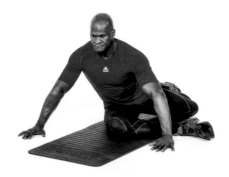

a

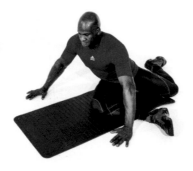

b

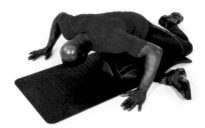

c

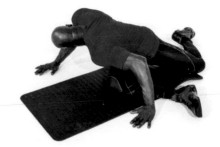

Photos 64 a-d   *d*

STARTING POSITION

Sit on the floor or on a mat with your knees bent at a 90-degree angle. Now rotate your trunk approximately 90 degrees so the trunk and the thigh toward which you are turning form a straight line. Hands are slightly more than shoulder-width apart on the floor.

EXECUTION

Lean toward the floor and continue to rotate your chest and pelvis until you feel a definite stretch. Hold this position for 20 to 30 seconds. Now return to the starting position, repeat the exercise, and then switch sides.

PLEASE NOTE:

As an alternative, the leg toward which you are turning can also be extended (hurdler's stretch).

PARTICIPATING MUSCLES

PRIMARY
Gluteus medius (m. gluteus medius)
Gluteus minimus (m. gluteus minimus)
Piriformis muscle (m. piriformis)

SECONDARY
External oblique muscle (m. obliquus externus abdominis)
Internal oblique muscle (m. obliquus internus abdominis)

M. SEMITENDINOSUS / M. BICEPS FEMORIS – THIGH MUSCLES

CLEAN AND JERK

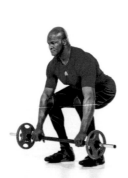

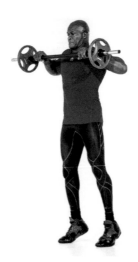

a

b

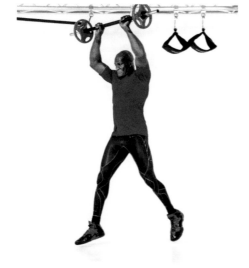

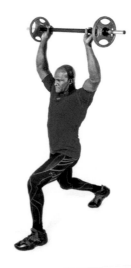

c

d

Photos 65 a-d

STARTING POSITION

Stand upright and bend your knees. Keep your back straight. Grip the barbell with hands shoulder-width apart, palms facing the floor.

EXECUTION

Keeping your back straight, lift the barbell to chin level. Next, engage your thigh muscles and pull the weight toward the chest while getting up on your toes. When the barbell is almost at chest level, switch your grip so your palms face the ceiling. At the same time jump up and thrust the weight overhead, landing in a lunge position.

PARTICIPATING MUSCLES

PRIMARY

Semitendinosus muscle (m. semitendinosus)
Biceps femoris muscle (m. biceps femoris)
Semimembranosus muscle (m. semimembranosus)

SECONDARY

Gastrocnemius muscle, lateral head (m. gastrocnemius, caput laterale)
Gastrocnemius muscle, medial head (m. gastrocnemius, caput mediale)
Gluteus medius (m. gluteus medius)
Gluteus maximus (m. gluteus maximus)
Vastus medialis muscle (m. vastus medialis)
Rectus femoris muscle (m. rectus femoris)
Vastus intermedius muscle (m. vastus intermedius)
Soleus muscle (m. soleus)

M. SEMITENDINOSUS / M. BICEPS FEMORIS – THIGH MUSCLES

LEG CURLS WITH ELASTIC BAND OR CABLE

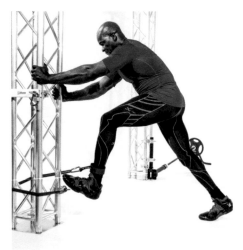

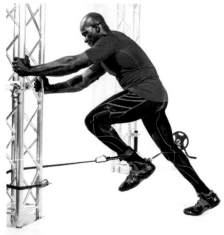

a

b

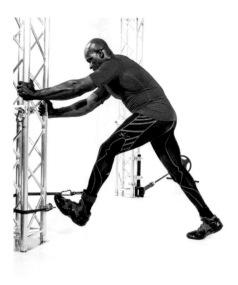

c

Photos 66 a-c

STARTING POSITION

Attach the band to your ankle with an ankle cuff. Hold on to a fixture in front of your body and plant the supporting leg as far back as possible, keeping a slanted body position. Arms are straight; the foot with the attached resistance is close to the attachment point.

EXECUTION

Now flex your knee and pull the heel back against the resistance. When the knee is fully bent slowly return to the starting position. Switch legs.

PLEASE NOTE:
Perform the motion slowly and keep the hip close to steady. Dorsal flexion of the ankle allows the calf muscles (m. gastrocnemius) to support knee flexion.

PARTICIPATING MUSCLES

PRIMARY
Semitendinosus muscle (m. semitendinosus)
Biceps femoris muscle (m. biceps femoris)
Semimembranosus muscle (m. semimembranosus)

SECONDARY
Gastrocnemius muscle, lateral head (m. gastrocnemius, caput laterale)
Gastrocnemius muscle, medial head (m. gastrocnemius, caput mediale)
Gluteus medius (m. gluteus medius)
Gluteus maximus (m. gluteus maximus)
Vastus medialis muscle (m. vastus medialis)
Rectus femoris muscle (m. rectus femoris)
Vastus intermedius muscle (m. vastus intermedius)
Soleus muscle (m. soleus)

M. SEMITENDINOSUS / M. BICEPS FEMORIS – THIGH MUSCLES

LEG CURLS WITH LARGE FITNESS BALL

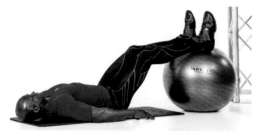

a

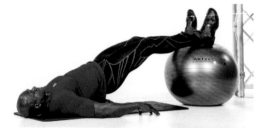

b

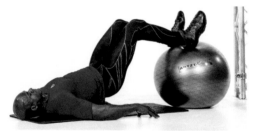

c

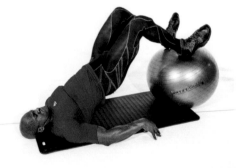

d

Photos 67 a-d

STARTING POSITION

Begin by lying on your back on the floor. Rest your lower legs on the fitness ball. Rest your arms on the floor alongside your body. Now straighten your knees and hips, lifting your lower back and hips off the floor.

EXECUTION

Once your hips are straight, bend your knees and pull your heels toward your posterior. Now only your heels should be on the ball. Straighten your knees again, return to the starting position, and repeat the exercise.

PLEASE NOTE:

Hips must remain straight during the movement. Dorsal flexion of the ankle decreases active insufficiency of the gastrocnemius, so it can contribute to knee flexion.

PARTICIPATING MUSCLES

PRIMARY

Biceps femoris muscle (m. biceps femoris)
Semitendinosus muscle (m. semitendinosus)
Semimembranosus muscle (m. semimembranosus)

SECONDARY

Gastrocnemius muscle, lateral head (m. gastrocnemius, caput laterale)
Gastrocnemius muscle, medial head (m. gastrocnemius, caput mediale)
Sartorius muscle (m. sartorius)
Gracilis muscle (m. gracilis)

M. SEMITENDINOSUS / M. BICEPS FEMORIS – THIGH MUSCLES

WHEEL LUNGE AGAINST RESISTANCE

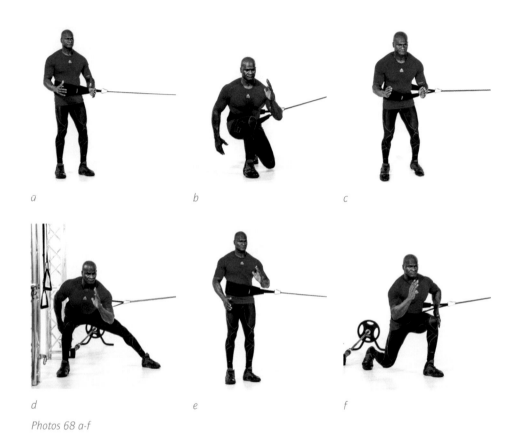

a   *b*   *c*

d   *e*   *f*

Photos 68 a-f

STARTING POSITION

Stand upright with legs hip-width apart. Arms are held loosely at hip level.

EXECUTION

Take a forward step. As you do so, flex the knee and hip until your back leg nearly touches the floor. Now return to the upright starting position.

Now take a diagonal step forward (approx. 45-degree angle) and return to the starting position. Finally take a sideways step. As you do so, flex the knee and the hip while keeping the supporting leg straight. Repeat each of these steps with the other leg.

PLEASE NOTE:
The chest is lifted, the abdomen muscles are engaged, and the shoulders are pulled back. Land softly, planting the heel of the forward foot. The forward knee should not jut out over the toes.

PARTICIPATING MUSCLES

PRIMARY
Rectus femoris muscle (m. recuts femoris)
Vastus lateralis muscle (m. vastus lateralis)
Vastus medialis muscle (m. vastus medialis)
Vastus intermedius muscle (m. vastus intermedius)
Semitendinosus muscle (m. semitendinosus)
Semimembranosus muscle (m. semimembranosus)
Biceps femoris muscle (m. biceps femoris)

SECONDARY
Gluteus medius (m. gluteus medius)
Gluteus maximus (m. gluteus maximus)
Long adductor muscle (m. adductor longus)
Short adductor muscle (m. adductor brevis)
Adductor magnus muscle (m. adductor magnus)
Gracilis muscle (m. gracilis)
Gastrocnemius muscle, medial head (m. gastrocnemius, caput mediale)
Gastrocnemius muscle, lateral head (m. gastrocnemius, caput laterale)
Soleus muscle (m. soleus)

M. SEMITENDINOSUS / M. BICEPS FEMORIS – THIGH MUSCLES

LATERAL JUMPS OVER OBSTACLE

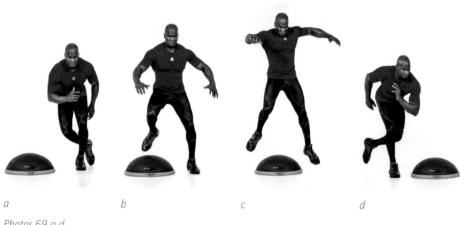

a   b   c   d

Photos 69 a-d

STARTING POSITION

Stand upright with legs hip-width apart. Elbows are bent and support the jumping motion.

EXECUTION

Get into a slight squat on one leg by flexing the knee, hip, and ankle. Immediately jump up and as far to the other side as you can, landing on the opposite foot. Repeat this exercise, alternating the jumping and landing leg.

PLEASE NOTE:

You will gather additional momentum if you swing your arms in rhythm with the movement. Lift your chest and engage your trunk muscles. To increase the degree of difficulty, decrease the amount of time between jumps.

PARTICIPATING MUSCLES

PRIMARY

Semitendinosus muscle (m. semitendinosus)

Semimembranosus muscle (m. semimembranosus)

Biceps femoris muscle (m. biceps femoris)

Adductor magnus muscle (m. adductor magnus)

Rectus femoris muscle (m. recuts femoris)

Vastus lateralis muscle (m. vastus lateralis)

Vastus medialis muscle (m. vastus medialis)

Vastus intermedius muscle (m. vastus intermedius)

Gracilis muscle (m. gracilis)

Gastrocnemius muscle, medial head (m. gastrocnemius, caput mediale)

Gastrocnemius muscle, lateral head (m. gastrocnemius, caput laterale)

Soleus muscle (m. soleus)

Tibialis posterior muscle (m. tibialis posterior)

Tibialis anterior muscle (m. tibialis anterior)

Gluteus medius (m. gluteus medius)

Gluteus minimus (m. gluteus minimus)

Tensor fasciae latae muscle (m. tensor fasciae latae)

SECONDARY

Rectus abdominis muscle (m. rectus abdominis)

Transverse abdominis (m. transversus abdominis)

Longissimus thoracis muscle (m. longissimus thoracis)

Multifidus muscle (m. multifidii)

External oblique muscle (m. obliquus externus abdominis)

Internal oblique muscle (m. obliquus internus abdominis)

M. GRACILIS – GRACILIS MUSCLE

SUPINE HIP ADDUCTION WITH ELASTIC RESISTANCE

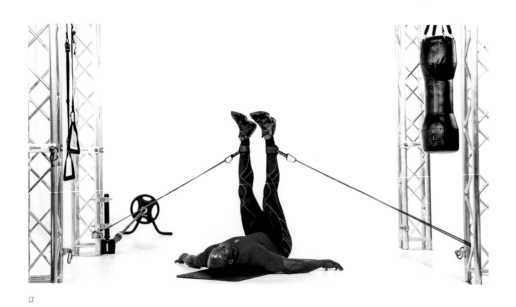

a

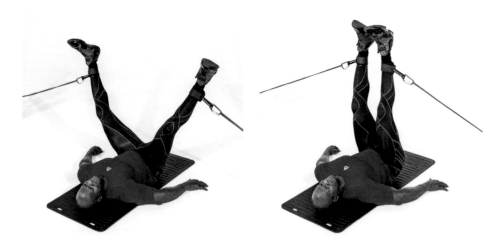

b

c

Photos 70 a-c

STARTING POSITION

Sit between two resistance bands (cables) and attach an ankle cuff to each ankle. Make sure your hips are between the two pulls. Now lie on your back and raise your legs in a vertical position.

EXECUTION

Move your legs into a straddle position until you feel a stretch. Close your legs and repeat the exercise.

PARTICIPATING MUSCLES

PRIMARY
Adductor magnus muscle (m. adductor magnus)
Short adductor muscle (m. adductor brevis)
Long adductor muscle (m. adductor longus)

SECONDARY
Pectinaeus muscle (m. pectinaeus)
Gracilis muscle (m. gracilis)

M. TENSOR FASCIAE LATAE – TENSOR FASCIAE LATAE MUSCLE

HIP ABDUCTION WITH ELASTIC RESISTANCE

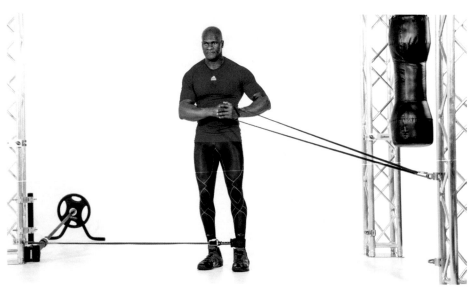

a

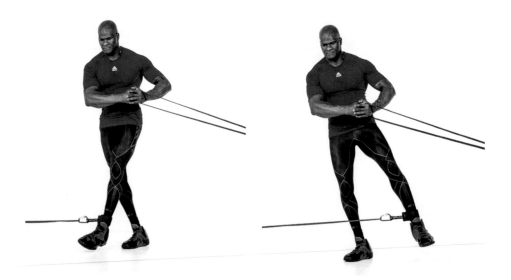

b   c

Photos 71 a-c

STARTING POSITION

Stand in front of the lower pull and attach the ankle cuff or band to your ankle. Now take a step back with the other leg and turn slightly to the side so the leg with the band attached to it is farther away from the pull than the other leg. To keep your balance, you can support yourself lightly against a grab pole or with the band. Stand on the leg that is closest to the pull. This allows the other leg to move in front of the supporting leg.

EXECUTION

Lift the leg with the resistance off the floor and first move it slightly to the inside (across the supporting leg). Now pull that leg to the outside as far as you can. The trunk does not move. Return to the starting position, repeat the exercise, and then switch legs.

PLEASE NOTE:

Make sure the band is attached as shown in the photo so the exercise can be performed correctly. You can support yourself with one or both arms, as is also shown.

PARTICIPATING MUSCLES

PRIMARY

Gluteus maximus (m. gluteus maximus)
Tensor fasciae latae muscle (m. tensor fasciae latae)
Gluteus minimus (m. gluteus minimus)

M. SOLEUS – CALF MUSCLES

SPLIT LUNGE JUMPS

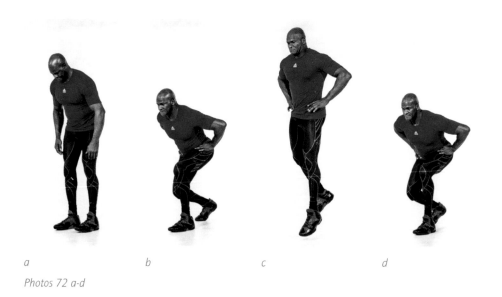

a   b   c   d

Photos 72 a-d

STARTING POSITION

Stand upright with legs hip-width apart and arms hanging at your sides. Take a forward step.

EXECUTION

Bend your knees and hips until the back knee touches the floor. Immediately jump up as high as you can. As you do so, keep your legs in lunge position. Land softly and return to the starting position. Repeat the exercise with the same leg. The forward knee should not jut out over the toes. After 10 jumps, switch legs and repeat the exercise on the other side.

PLEASE NOTE:
You will gather additional momentum if you swing your arms in rhythm with the movement. Lift your chest and engage your trunk muscles. To increase the degree of difficulty, decrease the amount of time between jumps.

PARTICIPATING MUSCLES

PRIMARY
Gluteus maximus (m. gluteus maximus)

Gluteus medius (m. gluteus medius)

Rectus femoris muscle (m. recuts femoris)

Vastus lateralis muscle (m. vastus lateralis)

Vastus medialis muscle (m. vastus medialis)

Vastus intermedius muscle (m. vastus intermedius)

Semitendinosus muscle (m. semitendinosus)

Semimembranosus muscle (m. semimembranosus)

Biceps femoris muscle (m. biceps femoris)

Gastrocnemius muscle, medial head (m. gastrocnemius, caput mediale)

Gastrocnemius muscle, lateral head (m. gastrocnemius, caput laterale)

Soleus muscle (m. soleus)

Achilles tendon

SECONDARY
Rectus abdominis muscle (m. rectus abdominis)

Transverse abdominis (m. transversus abdominis)

Longissimus thoracis muscle (m. longissimus thoracis)

Multifidus muscle (mm. multifidii)

Quadratus lumborum muscle (m. quadratus lumborum)

M. TIBIALIS ANTERIOR – TIBIALIS ANTERIOR MUSCLE

VERTICAL LEAP

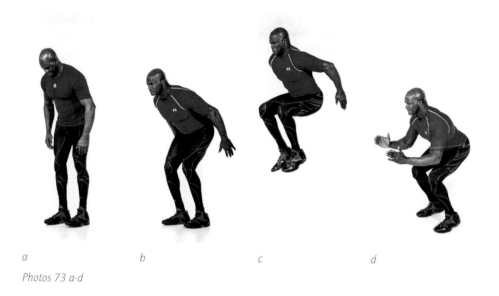

a   b   c   d

Photos 73 a-d

STARTING POSITION

Stand upright with legs hip-width apart and arms hanging at your sides.

EXECUTION

Get into a squat position by bending knees, hips, and ankles. Immediately jump as high as you can. Land softly and repeat the exercise.

PLEASE NOTE:

You will gather additional momentum if you swing your arms in rhythm with the movement. Lift your chest and engage your trunk muscles. To increase the degree of difficulty, decrease the amount of time between jumps.

PARTICIPATNG MUSCLES

PRIMARY
Gluteus maximus (m. gluteus maximus)

Semitendinosus muscle (m. semitendinosus)

Semimembranosus muscle (m. semimembranosus)

Biceps femoris muscle (m. biceps femoris)

Adductor magnus muscle (m. adductor magnus)

Rectus femoris muscle (m. rectus femoris)

Vastus lateralis muscle (m. vastus lateralis)

Vastus medialis muscle (m. vastus medialis)

Vastus intermedius muscle (m. vastus intermedius)

Gastrocnemius muscle, medial head (m. gastrocnemius, caput mediale)

Gastrocnemius muscle, lateral head (m. gastrocnemius, caput laterale)

Soleus muscle (m. soleus)

Achilles tendon

Tibialis anterior muscle (m tibialis anterior)

Extensor digitorum longus muscle (m. extensor digitorum longus)

SECONDARY
Deltoid muscle, anterior head (m. deltoideus, pars clavicularis)

Deltoid muscle, middle head (m. deltoideus, pars acromialis)

Supraspinatus muscle (m. supraspinatus)

Pectoralis major muscle, clavicular head (m. pectoralis major, pars clavicularis)

Biceps brachii (m. biceps brachii)

Trapezius muscle, lower fibers (m. trapezius, pars ascendens)

Trapezius muscle, middle fibers (m. trapezius, pars transversa)

Serratus anterior muscle (m. serratus anterior)

Rectus abdominis muscle (m. rectus abdominis)

M. RECTUS FEMORIS – RECTUS FEMORIS MUSCLE

MOUNTAIN CLIMBER

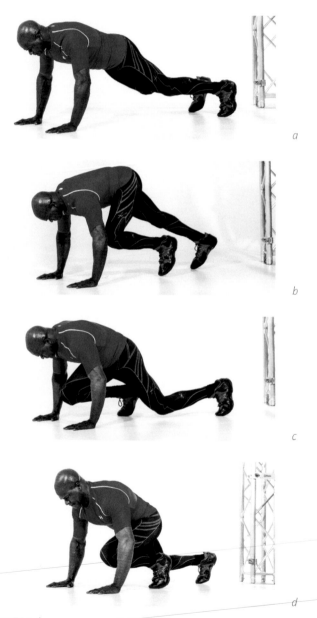

a

b

c

d

Photos 74 a-d

STARTING POSITION

Get down on all fours and then extend your legs back into a plank position.

EXECUTION

Now pull one leg forward toward the chest, and then extend it back again. Then immediately pull the other leg forward and extend it back.

PARTICIPATING MUSCLES

PRIMARY

Transverse abdominal muscle (m. transversus abdominis)

Rectus femoris muscle (m. rectus femoris)

Vastus lateralis muscle (m. vastus lateralis)

Vastus medialis muscle (m. vastus medialis)

Vastus intermedius muscle (m. vastus intermedius)

SECONDARY

Rectus abdominis muscle (m. rectus abdominis)

Gluteus medius (m. gluteus medius)

Gluteus maximus (m. gluteus maximus)

Deltoid muscle, anterior head (m. deltoideus, pars clavicularis)

M. VASTUS MEDIALIS/LATERALIS – INNER/OUTER THIGH MUSCLES
SUMO DEADLIFT WITH BARBELL

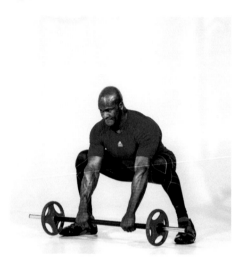

a

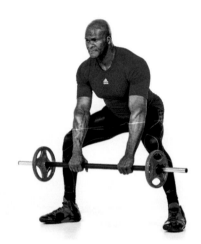

b

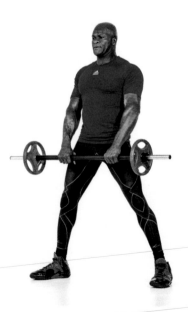

c

Photos 75 a-c

STARTING POSITION

Place your feet very far apart below the barbell. Now get into a squat position and using the palm grip, grip the bar between your legs with your hands shoulder-width apart or slightly closer together.

EXECUTION

Pull the barbell up by completely straightening the hips and knees. When the barbell has reached its highest position, pull your shoulders back. Return to the starting position and repeat the exercise.

PLEASE NOTE:

Keep your hips low, your shoulders up, and arms and legs straight when you lift. During the movement, the knees point in the same direction as the toes. To optimize the mechanical lever, keep the barbell close to the body as you pull it up.

PARTICIPATING MUSCLES

PRIMARY
Gluteus maximus (m. gluteus maximus)

SECONDARY
Rectus femoris muscle (m. rectus femoris)
Vastus medialis muscle (m. vastus medialis)
Vastus lateralis muscle (m. vastus lateralis)
Adductor magnus muscle (m. adductor magnus)
Soleus muscle (m. soleus)
Vastus intermedius muscle (m. vastus intermedius)

5.2 SYSTEMATIC COMPLEXITY – PILLARS AND PLANES

In this practice chapter we provide complex exercises that are performed largely with small pieces of equipment to promote complexity and optimize the transfer to everyday life. Here emphasis is placed on the pillars and planes concept. Get excited about the "best of Lamar" exercises that will highlight your individual limits and capabilities.

5.2.1 BAND AND PULLEY TRAINING I + II

There are different ways of attaching the bands to an external fixture, such as a door (door anchor), sturdy posts or handles, car doors, or with the help of a partner. Different degrees of difficulty can be achieved by attaching the bands at different heights (high, centrally, low). The active ends of the bands can be gripped with or without hand pulls or loops or can be attached at the waist.

I.   PULLING IN A STANDING POSITION (HIGH, MIDDLE, LOW)

Step progression:

1.   UPPER BODY ONLY

Both arms simultaneously ▸ alternating arms ▸ with upper body movement ▸ one arm only ▸ one arm with upper body movement

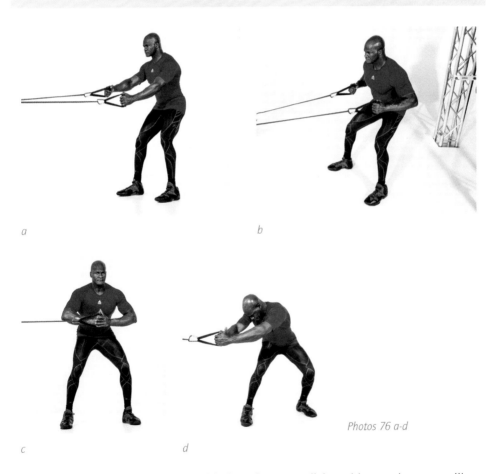

a

b

c

d

Photos 76 a-d

The pulling progression begins with legs in a parallel position and arms pulling simultaneously. One variation is to stand with your side to the attachment point, which activates multiple movement planes (sagittal, frontal, transverse).

2. UPPER AND LOWER BODY

Both arms simultaneously ▸ alternating arms ▸ one arm as well as parallel standing position ▸ lunge (small/big) ▸ on one leg

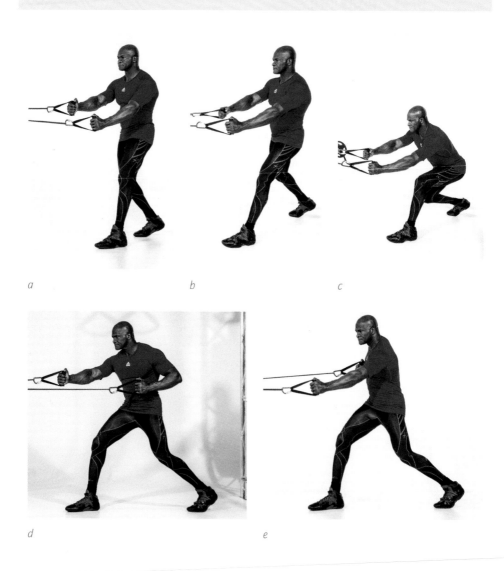

a   b   c

d   e

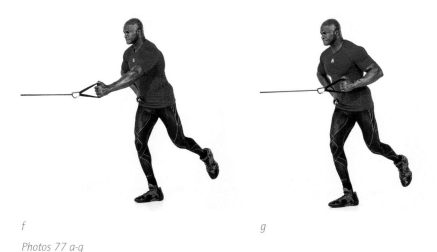

f   *g*

Photos 77 a-g

The lunge extends the base for pulling. A narrower base improves balance and, thus, makes the exercise easier. Gripping and pulling on one leg is one of the best exercise progressions to expand locomotion exercises.

3.   WHOLE BODY

Both arms simultaneously ▸ alternating arms ▸ with upper body movement ▸ one arm only ▸ one arm with upper body movement as well as parallel stance ▸ lunge (small/big) ▸ on one leg as well as upright ▸ bent over ▸ twisted ▸ combination ▸ stepping (sagittal plane, frontal plane, transverse plane)

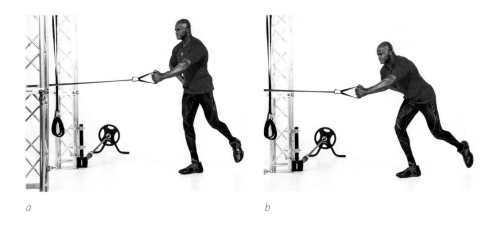

a   *b*

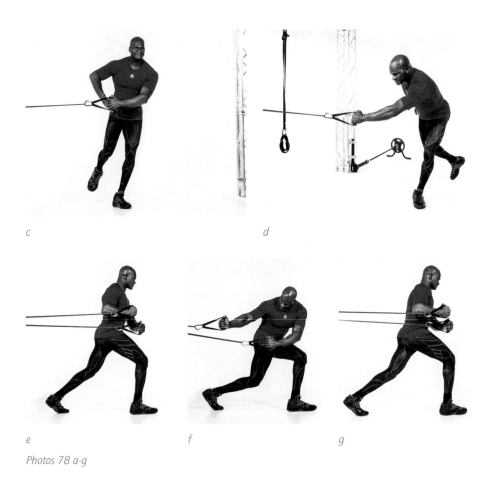

c

d

e

f

g

Photos 78 a-g

Pulling the band in a bent-over position makes the deceleration progression more challenging.

II. PRESSING IN A STANDING POSITION (HIGH, MIDDLE, LOW)

Step progression:

1. UPPER BODY ONLY

Both arms simultaneously ▸ alternating arms ▸ with upper body movement ▸ one arm only ▸ one arm with upper body movement

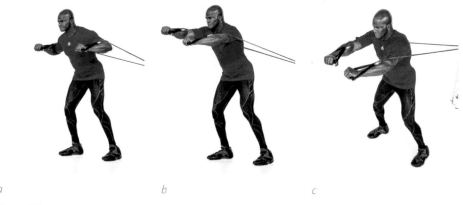

a   *b*   *c*

Photos 79 a-c

The pressing progression also begins with a parallel stance with simultaneous pressing.

2. UPPER AND LOWER BODY

Both arms simultaneously ▸ alternating arms ▸ one arm only as well as parallel stance ▸ lunge (small/big) ▸ on one leg

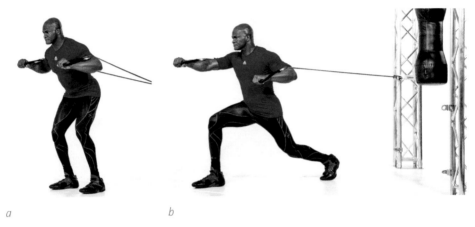

a   *b*

Photos 80 a-b

The lunge is the best position for working against resistance, but it requires more balance, particularly when using an alternating arm pattern for pressing.

When getting into the squat position or lunge, lean forward a little. Return the trunk to a vertical position during the standing-up phase.

3. WHOLE BODY

Both arms simultaneously ▸ alternating arms ▸ with upper body movement ▸ one arm only ▸ one arm with upper body movement as well as parallel stance ▸ lunge (small/big) ▸ on one leg as well as upright ▸ bent over [A] twisted ▸ combination ▸ stepping (sagittal plane, frontal plane, transverse plane)

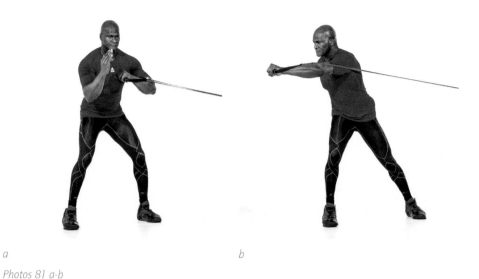

a   *b*

Photos 81 a-b

Stepping while pressing brings a dynamic quality to this whole-body progression.

5.2.2 FITNESS BALL TRAINING I + II

I. CHEST, SHOULDERS, BALANCE

CHEST

1. Push-up

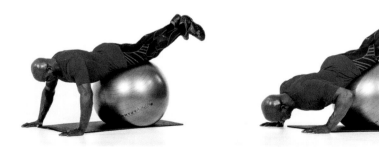

a   *b*

Photos 82 a-b

a) Both legs on the ball

b) One leg on the ball
Progression: hip support ▸ instep ▸ toes

c) Both hands on the ball, both feet on the floor
Progression: push up ▸ shift weight ▸ lift one leg

2. Arm jumps in prone position

Progression: hip support ▸ instep ▸ toes as well as varying the height and direction of the jumps (forward, backward, to the side)

SHOULDERS

A past weakness in fitness ball training was the shoulder work. There were no weight exercises with the ball that could simulate overhead presses with less than bodyweight. Until now!

1. Push-up variations

a) With bent knees
Bend the elbows and push up (photo 82, a-b).

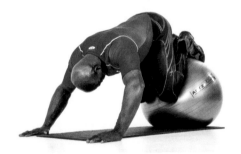 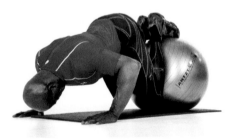

a   *b*

Photos 83 a-b

b) Pike press with extended legs
From the starting position of a, plant your toes and extend your legs all the way.
Now also bend the elbows and straighten them.

c) Pike press on one leg

Like b but with weight shifted to one leg; do push-ups in this position.

2. Rollercoaster (with two balls)

Lie with your chest on the ball and brace your feet against the floor. Hold another smaller ball between your knees. Roll on the ball into a push-up position while simultaneously lifting your bent knees that hold the second ball. Perform a push-up and immediately push back into the starting position.

BACK

The fitness ball allows you to target different muscles in the back—the small muscles that stabilize, as well as the large ones that are primarily responsible for movement.

1. Roll out

a) In a kneeling position, roll out to your shoulders with extended arms (first the arms, then the hips follow) (photo 83, a-b).

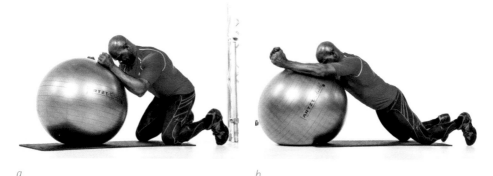

a   b

Photos 84 a-b

b) Like a, but start with legs extended (motion originates strictly from the arms). In addition, the ball can be used as an unstable environment (seat, support surface) for traditional back exercises (e.g., row with weights).

BALANCE, STRENGTH, AND STABILITY

Balance and stability training are basic components of working with the fitness ball. But you can also emphasize these elements individually by making them the main feature or limiting factor of an exercise. Here are a few examples:

1. Balance in a seated position by lifting legs, moving arms, or shifting body weight.

2. Use a four-point balance progression on knees and hands (photo 85).

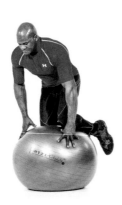
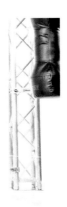

Photo 85

3. Use a two-point balance with knees on ball (photo 86).
Arm movements on different planes make the exercise more difficult.

Photo 86

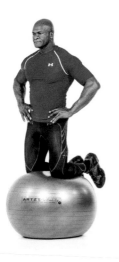

4. Use bounce training (shock lockouts).
From an upright position in front of the ball let yourself fall straight down (trunk muscle tension) onto the ball in front of you and stabilize this position. This exercise can be combined with push-up variations as acyclical bounce training.

II. LEGS, HIPS, AND TRUNK

LEGS AND HIPS

1. Gliding at the wall

Gliding exercises at the wall are a great way to prepare for intensive leg work or to strengthen the lower body. Gliding exercises can be used by anyone to strengthen legs in a functional and progressive way.

a) With your back to the wall
Progression: with two legs ▸ with one leg ▸ with one leg and the free leg extended

b) Facing the wall
Progression: with two legs ▸ with one leg

c) With your side to the wall
Progression: with two legs ▸ with the outside/inside leg

2. Squat
a) Backward with one leg from instep to toes (photo 87, a-f)
Progression: with different foot positions ▸ while moving with contralateral dynamic arm movement

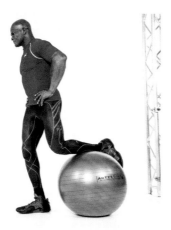 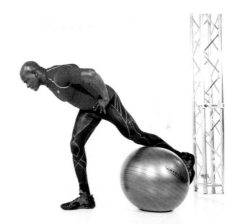

a   *b*

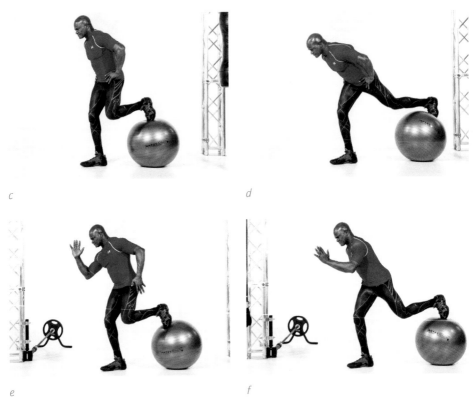

c

d

e

f

Photos 87 a-f

b) Sideways with one leg (photo 88, a-b)

Progression: with different foot positions legs ▸ with dynamic arm movement ▸ with leg circles or figure eights

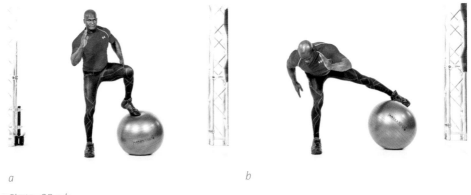

a

b

Photos 88 a-b

Glide and squat exercises can also be done with added weight.

HIPS (LUMBAR REGION)

1. Bridge variations

On your back with calves on the ball, lift and lower your hips.

Progression: both legs ▸ one leg ▸ only heels resting on ball ▸ movement

2. Trunk extension

a) Knees touch the floor; draped over the ball, lift your upper body.

b) Feet touch the floor; draped over the ball, lift your upper body (photo 89, a-b).

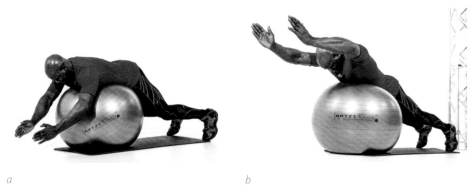

a   *b*

Photos 89 a-b

c) Contralateral superman (photo 90, a-b)

Whole-body extension in quadruped position; extend and one arm and the opposite leg and hold this position.

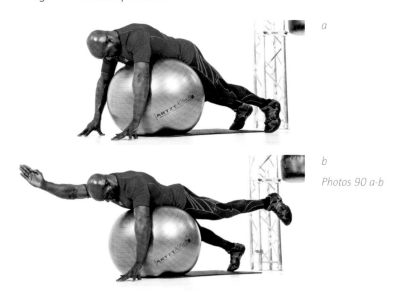

a

b

Photos 90 a-b

3. Leg raise

Draped over the ball on your back, raise both legs (vary arm positions).

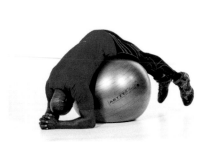 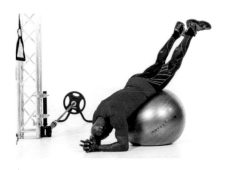

a   *b*

Photos 91 a-b

HIPS (ABDOMINALS/OBLIQUES)

1. Leg scissors

Twists with the ball

Progression: range of motion ▸ motion speed

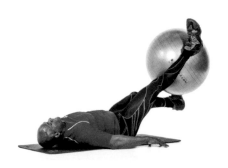 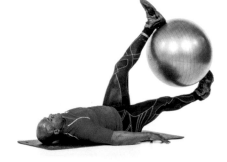

a   *b*

Photos 92 a-b

2. Downward-facing knee bends

Progression: foot position ▸ contact area ▸ both legs ▸ one leg ▸ one leg with additional free leg movement

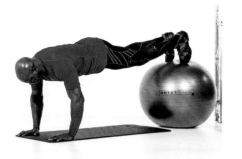
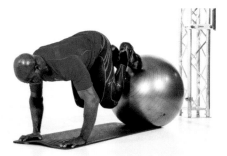

a   *b*

Photos 93 a-b

3. Pike press (see Shoulders)

4. Hip rollout (see Back)

5. Hip twist

From a push-up position, twist from the left leg to the right leg.

Progression: support surface ▸ range of motion ▸ speed ▸ inclined positions

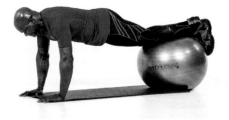

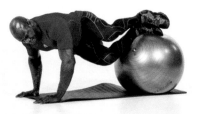

a   *b*

Photos 94 a-b

ABDOMINALS/OBLIQUES

Crunches

a) On your back with calves on the ball, raise your trunk.

b) 90-degree abdominal crunch (photo 95, a-c)

c) Reverse crunch like a, but lift the ball with your legs.

d) Side crunch with hip on the ball and legs extended and open (scissor position) by raising your trunk.

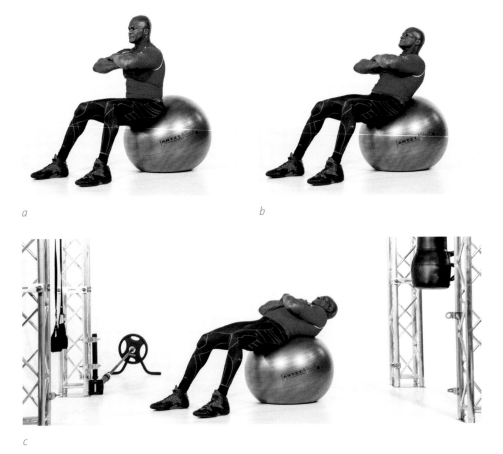

a

b

c

Photos 95 a-c

5.2.3 STROOPS AND STIK

The resistance bands that are outfitted with carabiner clips (Stroops) can be easily attached to sturdy posts or wall bars, and, together with the Fit Stik, create an ideal training tool for your plane training. Here, too, as with the band and pulley, you can achieve different degrees of difficulty when attaching the Stroops at varying heights (high, middle, low). Our theme continues to be pillars and planes. As a reminder:

THE FOUR PILLARS OF HUMAN MOVEMENT
Pillar 1: Standing and moving.
Pillar 2: Changing the plane of the center of gravity.
Pillar 3: Pulling and pushing.
Pillar 4: Rotation—directional change and torque.

THE THREE PLANES OF HUMAN MOVEMENT
❭ The vertical plane divides us into a right and left side.
❭ The frontal plane divides us into front and back.
❭ The horizontal plane is the plane of rotation that separates top from bottom.

I.   STROOPS AND STICK HIGH MOUNT

1. Lift/chop
Lunge position ▸ pull back to front with contralateral arm ▸ a) high ▸ b) middle ▸ c) low

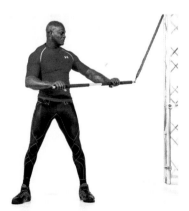

Photos 96

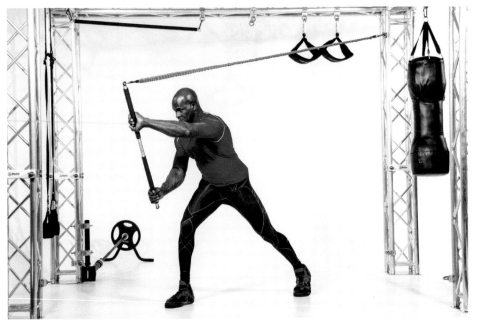

a

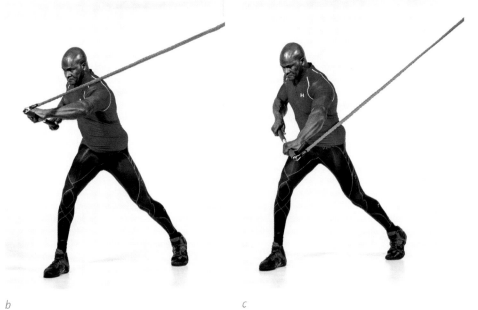

b   *c*

Photos 96 a-c

II. STROOPS AND STIK MIDDLE MOUNT

1. Circles/rotations

Wide lunge position ▸ arm circles ▸ rotation in both directions possible

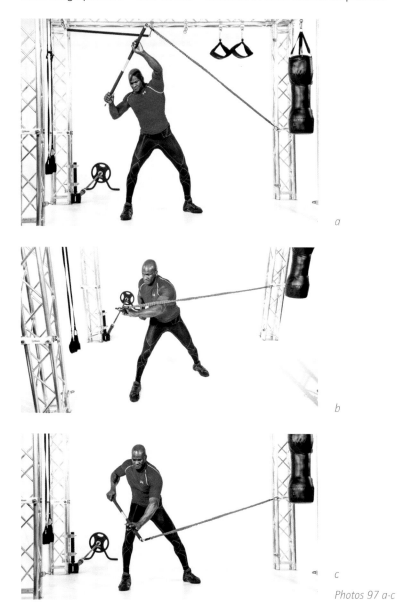

a

b

c

Photos 97 a-c

III. STROOPS AND STIK LOW MOUNT

1. Row

Lunge position ▸ leg movement/changing the lunge position ▸ pull the Fit Stik laterally past the body or forward

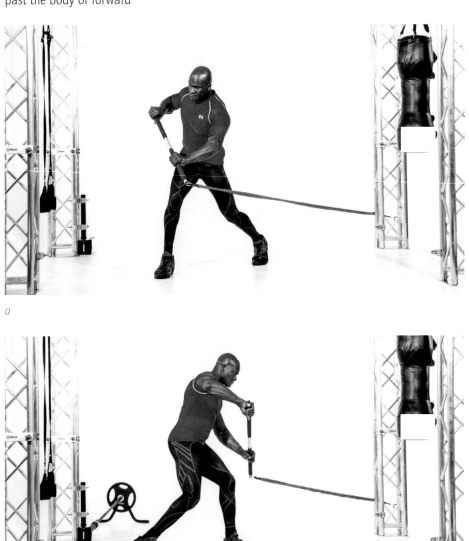

a

b

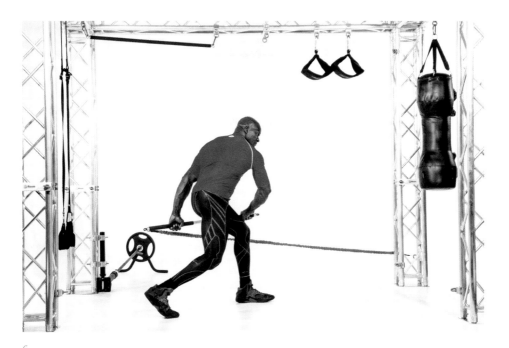

c

Photos 98 a-c

2. Lunge variation

Lunge position ▶ knee bend in lunge position holding the Stik (hold horizontal, contralateral) ▶ antirotation movement

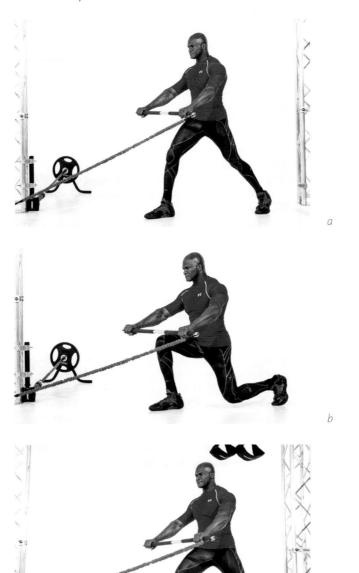

a

b

c

Photos 99 a-c

5.2.4 SLING TRAINING

The following sling trainer exercises are particularly challenging in coordination training. The additional instability provided by the deflection roller system used here can add maximum training stimuli.

I. FORWARD

1. Arm push

Push-up position ▸ hands in the loops and feet on the floor ▸ lunge with simultaneous arm push, contralateral

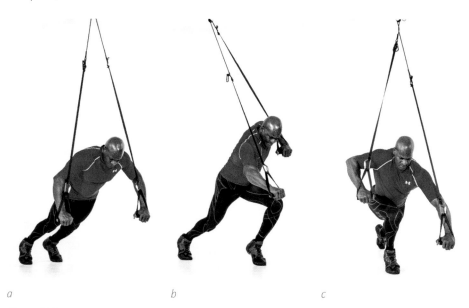

a   b   c

Photos 100 a-c

2. Extension

Push-up position ▸ hands in the loops and feet on the floor ▸ widen the arm–trunk angle from 90 degrees to 180 degrees by extending the arms forward

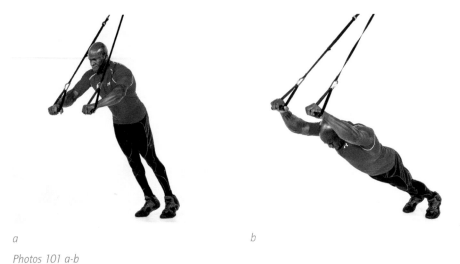

a   b

Photos 101 a-b

II. REVERSE

1. Pull-up

On your back, feet flat on the floor ▸ reverse pull-up ▸ pelvic lift into candle position

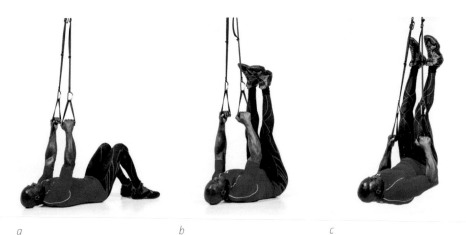

a   b   c

Photos 102 a-c

2. Pistol squat/knee bend

Body is on a slant, hands in loops ▸ shift weight to one leg, lift the free leg ▸ single-leg squat

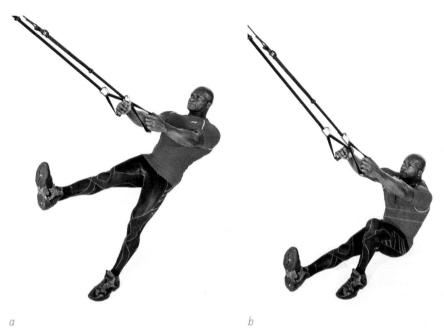

a

b

Photos 103 a-b

III. LATERAL

1. Trunk lift

Standing position, arms extended overhead ▶ lateral trunk lift

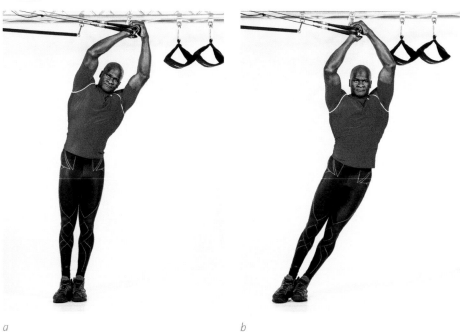

a   *b*

Photos 104 a-b

5.2.5 CORE TRAINER

The following exercises with the core trainer, which is essentially an Olympic bar (approx. 44 lbs.), focus primarily on strength.

I recommend the following exercises only for advanced clients with substantial core strength.

I. V-GRIP EXERCISES

1. Shoulder press

Standing position ▸ grip the bar with the right hand ▸ hoist, and with the left hand grip one side of the v-grip ▸ lift the bar higher and switch the right hand to the v-grip ▸ straighten the elbows

Always use this technique when the exercise begins with a hold in front of the body (high).

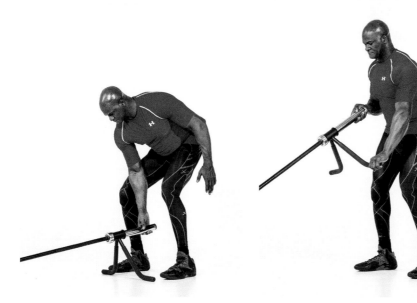

a   *b*

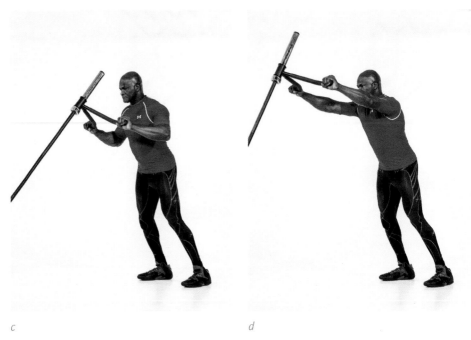

c

d

Photos 105 a-d

2. Twisted push, standing

Wide stance next to the bar ▸ rotate, opening into a lunge ▸ simultaneously push the bar up > foot turns to follow

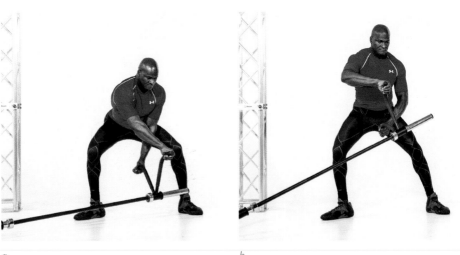

a

b

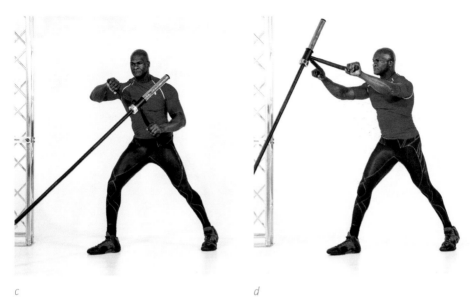

c   *d*

Photos 106 a-d

3. Reverse push, 180 degrees, standing

Stand with legs shoulder-width apart next to the bar with your back to the mount ▸ turn
180 degrees (back lunge, open up to the side, open forward into lunge position) and push
up

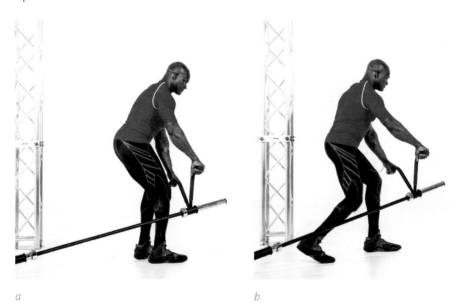

a   *b*

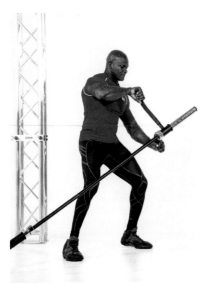

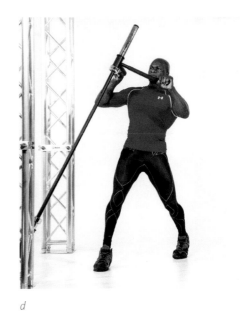

c

d

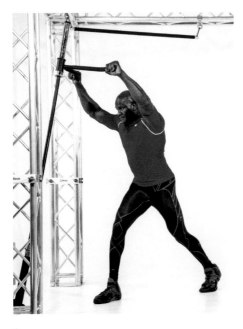

e

Photos 107 a-e

4. Twisted push with alternating legs in supine position

On your back, lift your feet, extend your arms ▸ rotate lower body (legs) to the right ▸ simultaneously extend the upper leg (left) ▸ when turning back onto the back bend the knee again and push the bar up ▸ switch sides

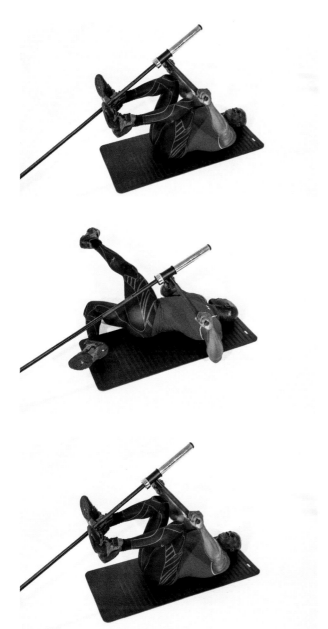

a

b

c

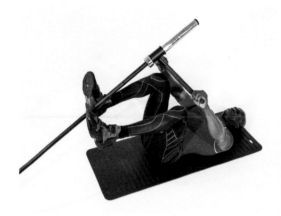

d

Photos 108 a-d

5. Twist in supine position

On your back with heels on the floor, arms extended ▸ rotate lower body (legs) to the right ▸ simultaneously move the bar to the left, moving elbows toward the floor ▸ knees remain closed ▸ switch sides

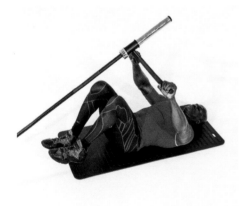
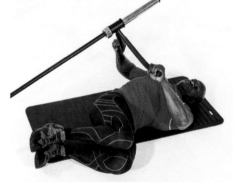

a   *b*

Photos 109 a-b

II. JACKHAMMER GRIP EXERCISES

1. Squat – push – rotation

Stand with feet shoulder-width apart and hold the bar at chest level ▸ squat ▸ push the bar up while simultaneously straightening your body (on your toes) ▸ rotate the bar left and downward while simultaneously bending your knees, the foot also turns ▸ stay low and move the bar to the right side ▸ with the bar at chest level, push up again and now rotate right

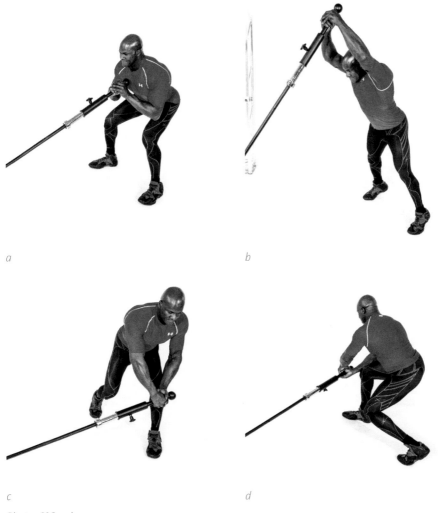

a

b

c

d

Photos 110 a-d

2. Upper cuts

Stand with feet shoulder-width apart and hold the bar at chest level ▸ perform upper cuts to the right and left

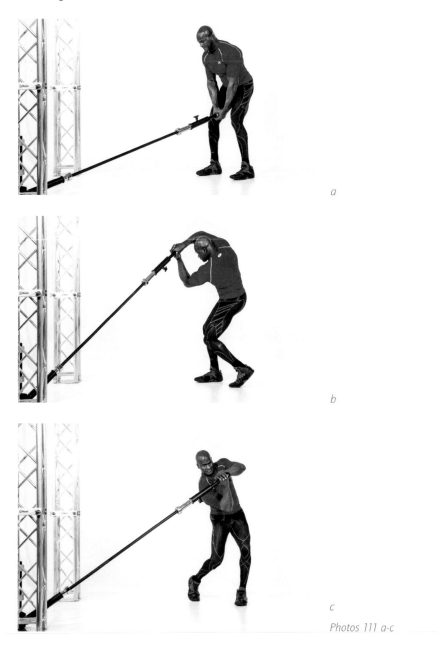

a

b

c

Photos 111 a-c

3. Single-arm clean and jerk

Stand with feet shoulder-width apart, bend your knees, hold the bar at shoulder level with your right hand, place the free hand on your hip ▸ do an explosive single-arm clean and jerk ▸ contralateral execution ▸ final position is a lunge

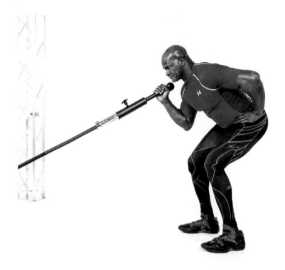

a

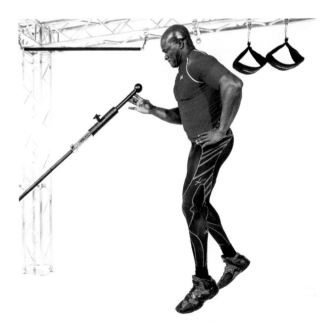

b

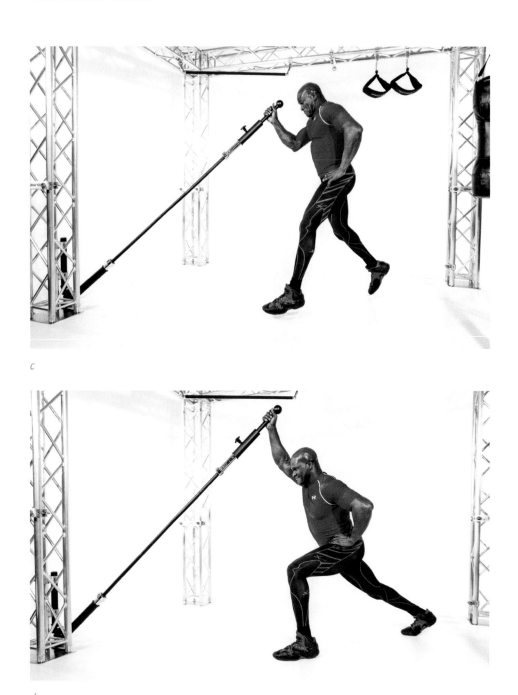

c

d

Photos 112 a-d

4. Push from a deep squat

Stand next to the bar with feet shoulder-width apart ▸ deep squat ▸ from the squat push upward on a diagonal ▸ continue to stand sideways, the leg turning to follow

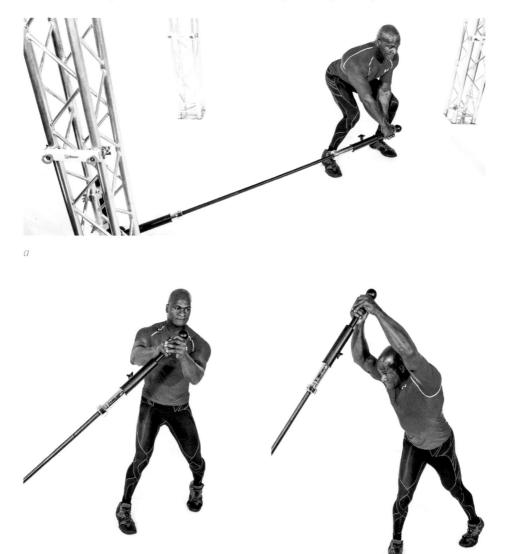

a

b

c

Photos 113 a-c

5. Y move

Stand with feet shoulder-width apart and hold the bar at chest level ▸ push up and to the right > come back to the center (chest level) > push up and to the left ▸ no leg movement

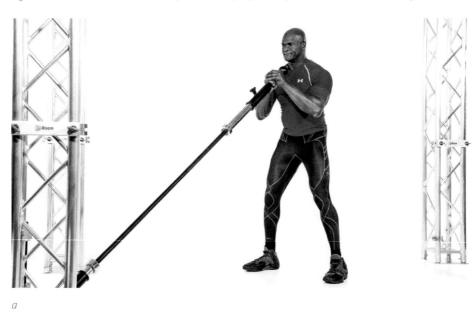

a

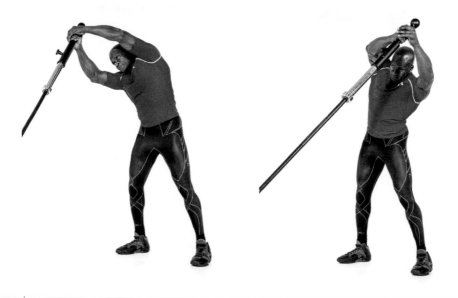

b   c

Photos 114 a-c

II. DOUBLE GRIP EXERCISES

1. Push

Stand with feet shoulder-width apart and hold the bar at knee level ▸ push the bar up ▸ leg moves back (lunge position)

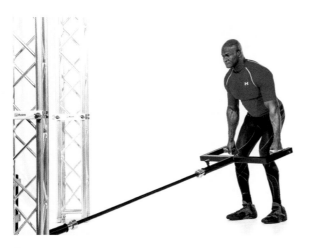
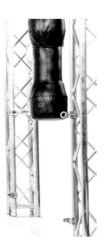

a

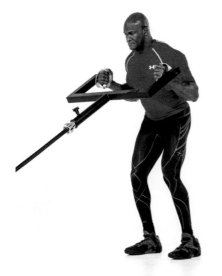
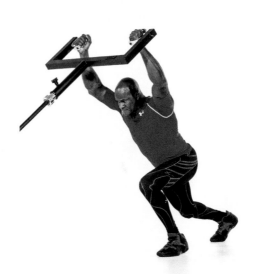

b *c*

Photos 115 a-c

2. Lateral steps

Stand with feet shoulder-width apart and hold the bar at knee level ▸ lateral step left, grip rotation (elbow flexion and arm adduction) ▸ final position is a squat ▸ switch sides

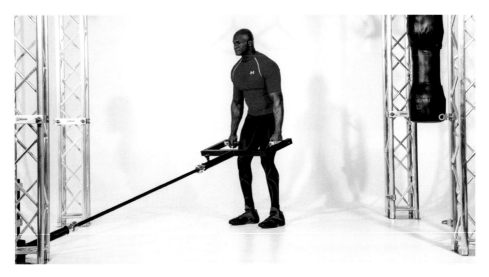

a

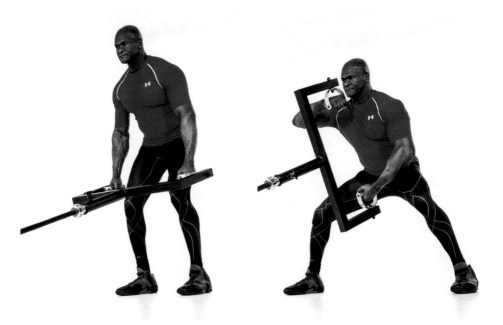

b   *c*

Photos 116 a-c

3. Biceps curls

Lunge, hold bar at knee level ▸ biceps curls

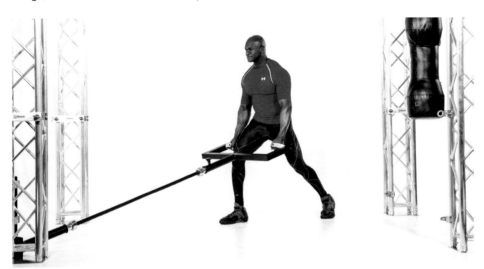

a

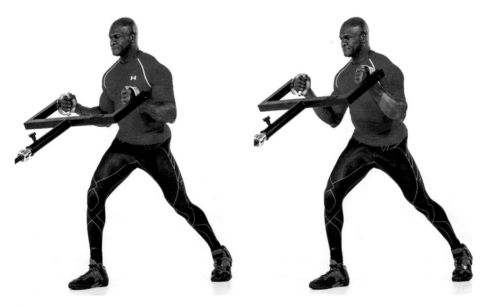

b   c

Photos 117 a-c

III. DOUBLE GRIP EXERCISES WITH BALLAST BALL

1. Push press

On your back, the bar at chest level, elbows are bent ▸ push the bar up ▸ shoulder blades stay on the ball

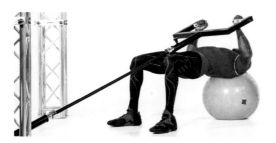

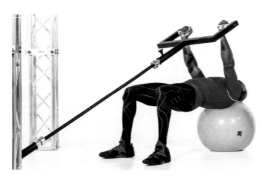

a

b

Photos 118 a-b

2. Diagonal push press

In a deep squat, push your back against the ball, elbows are bent, the bar is at chest level ▸ push the bar up and forward

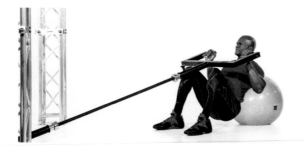
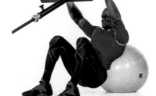

a

a

Photos 119 a-b

242

5.2.6 LARGE SLINGS

The following exercises are particularly challenging to trunk and arm strength and focus on rotation and directional changes.

1. Windshield wiper

Hang from the loops ▸ elbows at right angles ▸ do leg circles (right-left)

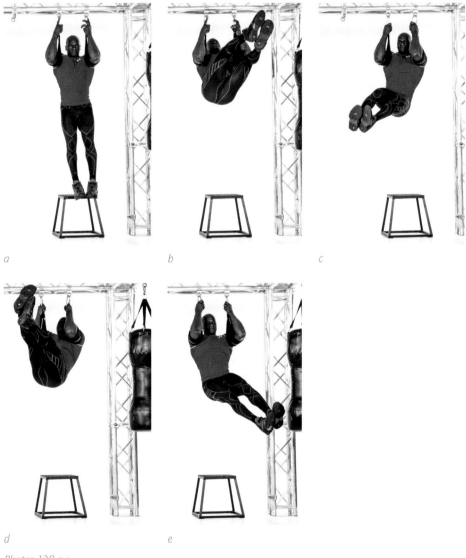

a   *b*   *c*

d   *e*

Photos 120 a-e

2. Scissors

Hang from the loops ▸ elbows at right angles ▸ do crossover scissors with legs

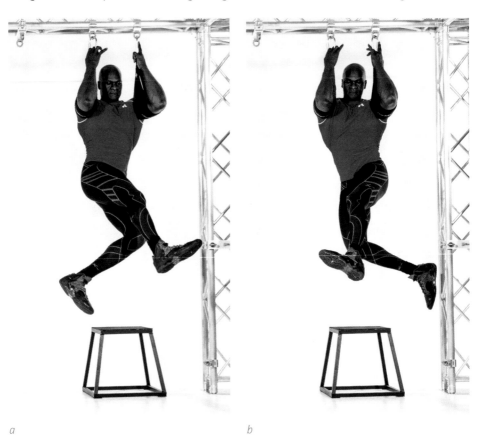

a   b

Photos 121 a-b

5.2.7 PUNCHING BAG

The following exercises with the punching bag are very advanced and require a lot of coordination.

1. Power-ups
Stand with your feet shoulder-width apart ▸ hold the bag above shin level ▸ hoist in front ▸ rotate ▸ rest it on your shoulder ▸ lower and switch sides

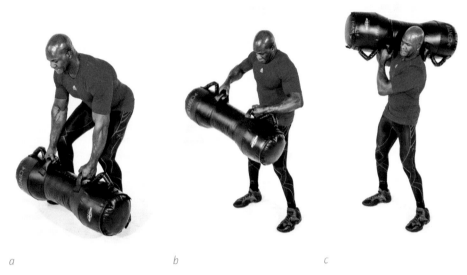

a   b   c

Photos 122 a-c

2. Power-ups clean and jerks

Back lunge ▸ hold the bag above shin level ▸ clean and jerk with shoulder press ▸ switch legs

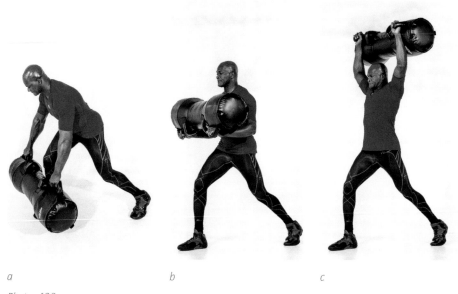

a   b   c

Photos 123 a-c

3. Push press

With your back on the ball, the bag at chest level, elbows bent ▸ push the bag up and back
▸ shoulder blades stay on the ball

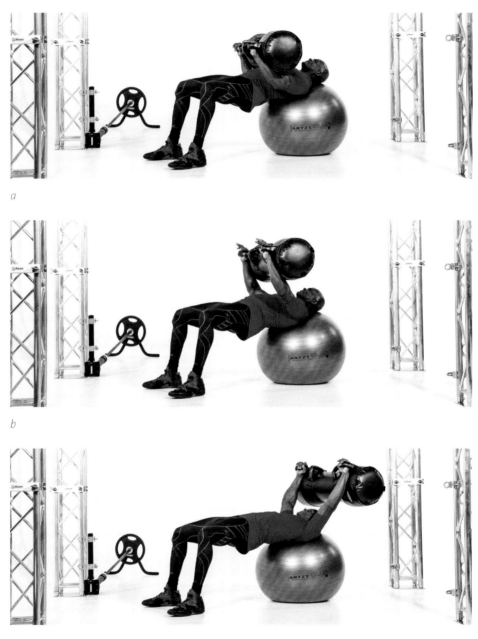

a

b

c

Photos 124 a-c

4. Push press on a slant

Deep squat with back against the ball, elbows bent ▸ push the bag up

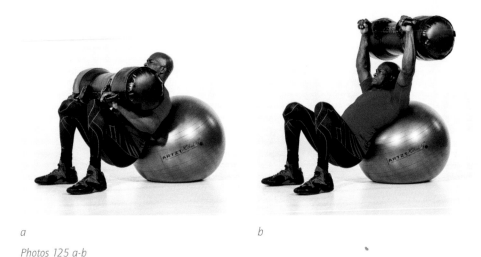

a   b

Photos 125 a-b

5. Y moves

Stand with feet shoulder-width apart ▸ from a shoulder-level position, alternately push the bag to the right and the left ▸ no leg movement

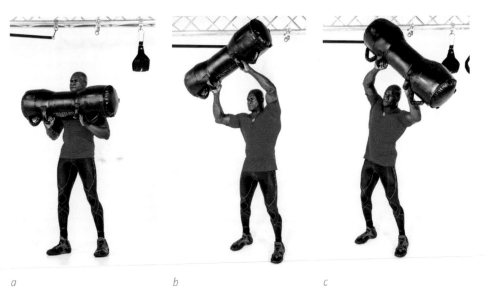

a   b   c

Photos 126 a-c

5.2.8 CORE BALL AND ELASTIC BAND

These exercises also require a lot of coordination.

1. Push variations

Lunge ▸ push forward (low, center, high) ▸ both arms simultaneously ▸ alternate arms ▸ with upper body movement ▸ with dynamic lunging movement (legs)

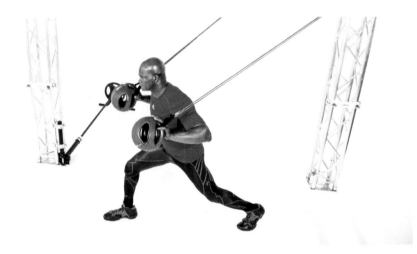

a

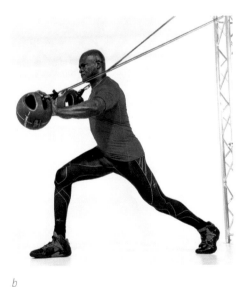

b

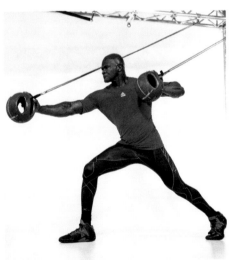

c

Photos 127 a-c

2. Butterfly

Lunge ▸ frontal butterfly arm movement ▸ with dynamic lunging movement (legs)

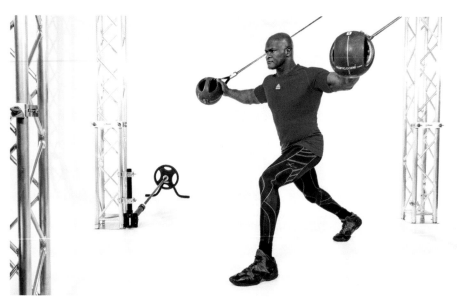

a

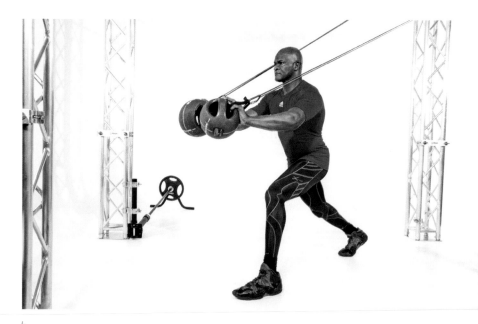

b

Photos 128 a-c

3. Overhead pull

Lunge with arms extended overhead ▸ pulling the bands from behind, move the arms downward ▸ use dynamic leg movement to move from an upright position into a lunge

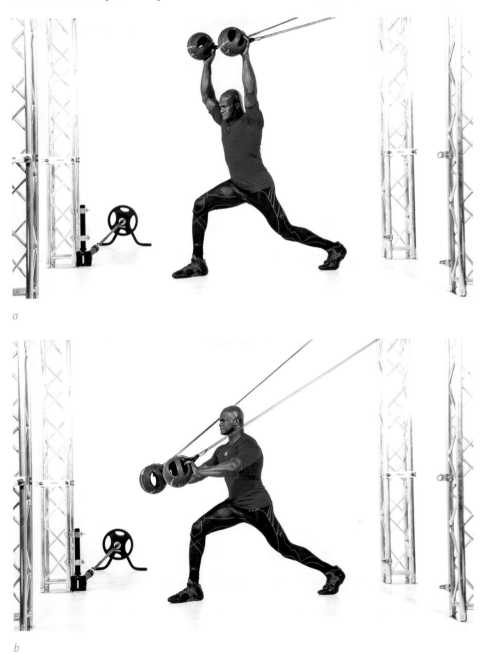

a

b

Photos 129 a-c

4. Backward pull

Stand with feet shoulder-width apart, knees slightly bent, arms extended in front of the body ▶ arm pull from the top, down, and back

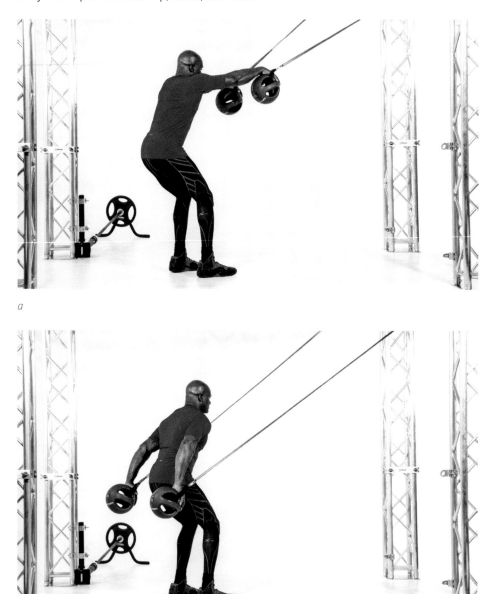

a

b

Photos 130 a-c

5. Diagonal pull

Stand with your side to the ball, the hand closest to the ball holds the ball, the arm is extended ▸ pull from the top down (across the front) ▸ combine with dynamic crossover step ▸ switch sides

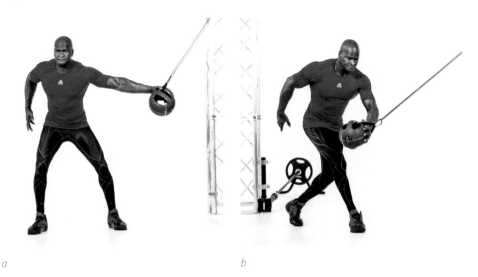

a   *b*

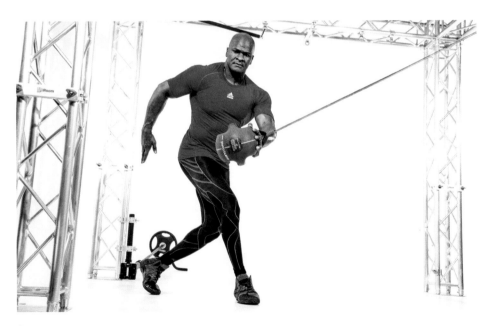

c

Photos 131 a-c

5.2.9 CORE BAR AND ELASTIC BAND

BALANCE, COORDINATION, AND LATERAL MOVEMENT

1. Dynamic push-up with static bar

Push-up position on the bar ▸ perform push-up without moving the bar up and down (only the body moves) ▸ watch your breath

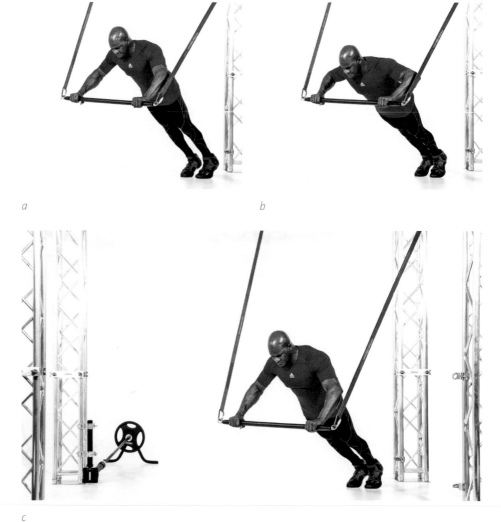

a

b

c

Photos 132 a-c

2. Dynamic push-up

Push-up position on the bar ▸ perform push-up without moving the body up and down (only the bar moves) ▸ watch your breath

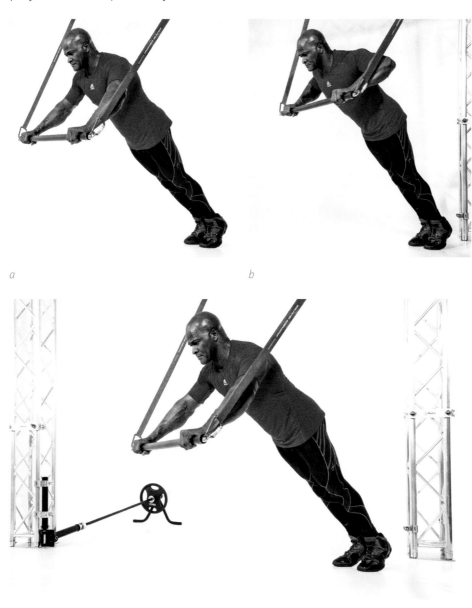

a   *b*

c

Photos 133 a-c

3. Dynamic lunge

Narrow stance, core bar in front of the body, wide grip ▶ lunge forward ▶ push with diagonal ipsilateral rotation

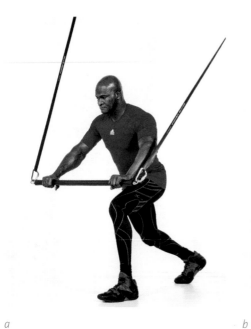

a

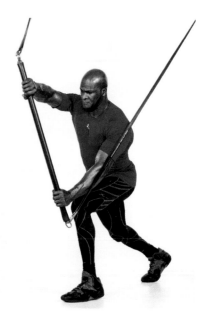

b

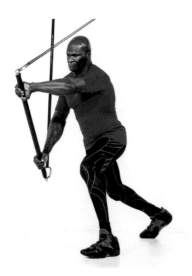

c

Photos 134 a-c

4. Split jerk

Stand with the band pulley from behind ▸ hold the bar at chest level ▸ push the bar from chest to shoulder level ▸ (a-c) lunge and simultaneously push the bar overhead ▸ (d-e) take a very dynamic big forward lunge and simultaneously push the bar forward and up

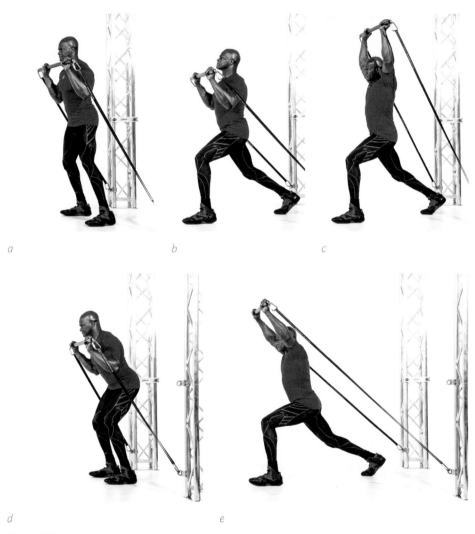

a   *b*   *c*

d   *e*

Photos 135 a-e

Another alternative is using a loose band and attaching it low or in the middle. The band should be gripped from behind with one hand ▸ squat ▸ lunge ▸ extend the arm with the band forward and up

5.2.10 ROPES

Along with the rope training we are familiar with from athletic training you can also use ropes very effectively as a flexible pull-up bar. These exercises are particularly well suited for advanced clients and focus primarily on core and power.

I. PARALLEL DOUBLE ROPE/VERTICAL PLANE

1. Backward roll

Hang from the ropes using a neutral grip ▸ roll backward 360 degrees ▸ lunge ▸ knees bent or straight

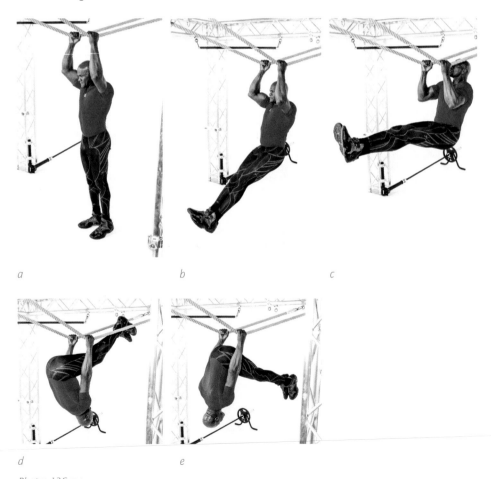

a　　　　　　　　*b*　　　　　　　　*c*

d　　　　　　　　*e*

Photos 136 a-e

2. Explosive pull-up

Jump up and grip the ropes to hang using a neutral grip ▸ pull up explosively while looking up and releasing the grip in the highest position ▸ grip again ▸ look up again and repeat

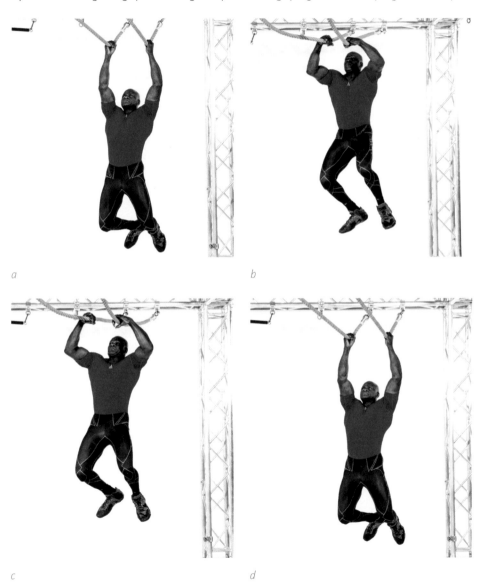

a

b

c

d

Photos 137 a-d

II. PARALLEL DOUBLE ROPE/FRONTAL PLANE

Pull-up

Hang from the ropes ▸ pull up while looking up ▸ knees bent or straight ▸ repeat

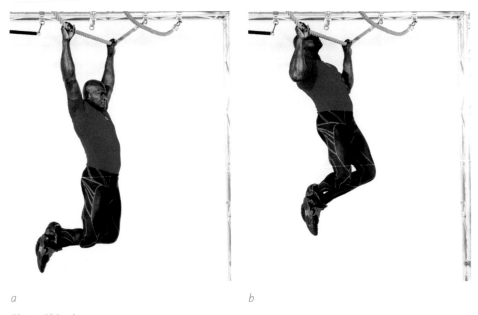

a   b

Photos 138 a-b

III. VERTICAL HANGING ROPE

Pull-up with offset hands

Grip the rope with hands in offset position, lift the lower body ▸ bend the elbows to 90 degrees and remain in static position ▸ bicycle the legs

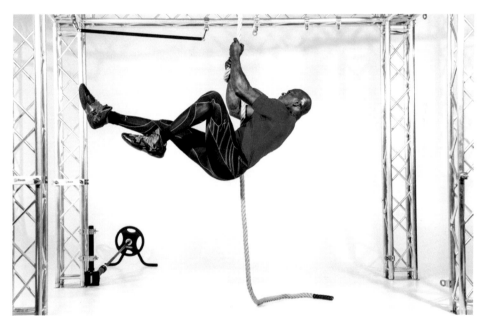

a

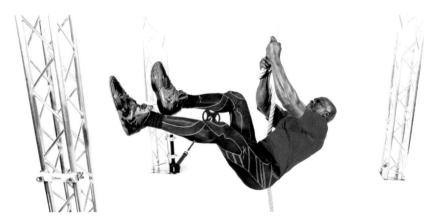

b

Photos 139 a-b

5.2.11 WEIGHTED BALL AND CONES

This final exercise sequence continues to focus on planes, but in the process you will work on changing the planes of the body's center of gravity. Here the changing planes refers to movements of the trunk and the lower extremities (or a combination of the two) that raise or lower the body's center of gravity. This complex exercise requires dexterity and mobility, aerobic fitness, speed and explosiveness, balance, strength (pushing and pulling), muscle endurance, reaction, and mental fitness.

180-degree push-and-pull circle

Front-facing stance, weighted ball in one hand (contralateral) ▸ push the ball successively (right to left and vice versa) toward the cones ▸ pull the ball back and push it toward the next cone ▸ change direction at the end ▸ call out changes in sequence

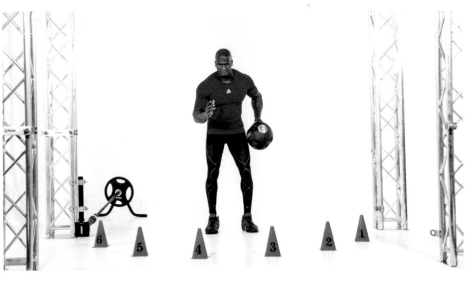

a

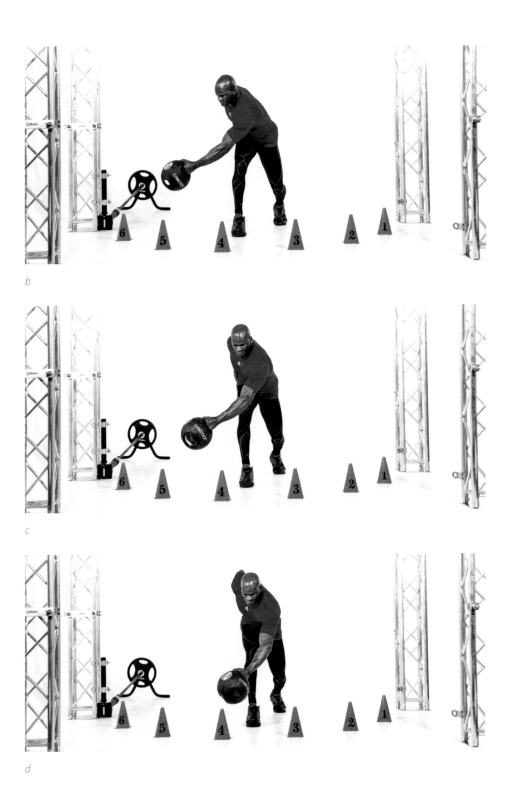

b

c

d

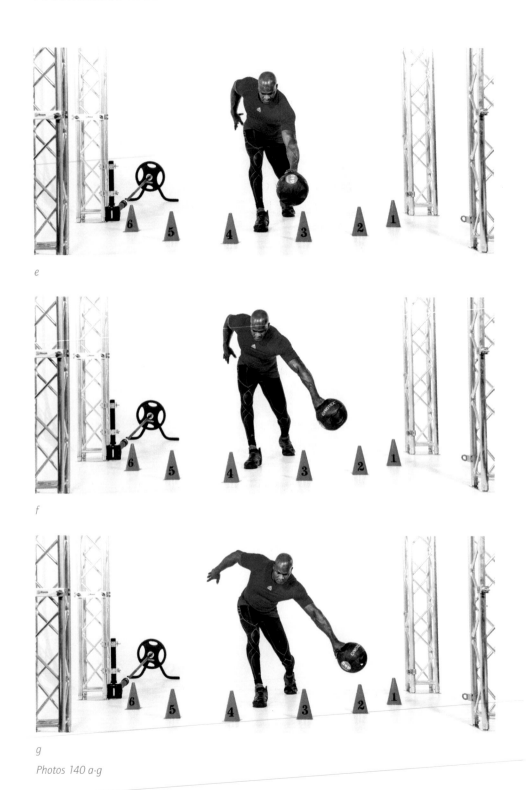

e

f

g

Photos 140 a-g

5.3 CIRCUIT TRAINING AND WORKOUTS

The following programs are combinations of exercises from chapter 5. When combining these exercises, I was particularly concerned with the functional and holistic concept. All programs are designed to offer functional whole-body workouts that can be performed by beginners as well as advanced exercisers (with the exception of the core trainer circuit). As previously mentioned at the beginning of chapter 5, the dosage must be customized for individual clients—their goals and habits. It is the only way the following circuit training can be successful long term.

Levels 1, 2, and 3 with the corresponding sets are comparable to the training statuses listed on pages 95 and 96.

Level 1 = Beginner (unfit)

Level 2 = Recreational athlete/intermediate (moderately fit)

Level 3 = Athlete/advanced (fit)

But you must make sure that the chosen programs contain exercises from chapter 5.2, Systematic Complexity. An absolute beginner should, therefore, revert to the basics (chapter 5.1) and only start with level 1 circuit training after he has established a solid fitness foundation. Here it is your job as a trainer to facilitate an optimal start and effective training structure for your clients. Remember that small pieces of fitness equipment often add to the progression or increase of coordination requirements in an exercise and that their suitability is, therefore, limited for beginner use.

LAMAR SYSTEM WORKOUT 1

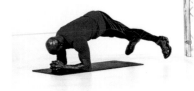

1. Plank jacks

30 repetitions

See pg. 158, photo 55, a-c

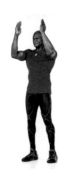

2. Bent-over row

15 repetitions

See pg. 116, photo 34, a-b

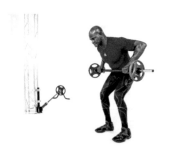

3. Pullover

25 repetitions

See pg. 144, photo 48, a-d

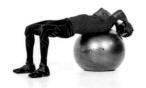

4. Shoulder 90 degrees dynamic

20 repetitions

See pg. 130, photo 41, a-d

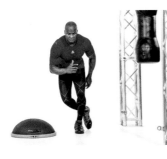

5. **Lateral jumps over obstacle**
20 repetitions
See pg. 186, photo 69, a-d

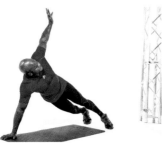

6. **T push-up**
20 repetitions
See pg. 152, photo 52, a-b

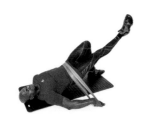

7. **Hip extension with elastic band**
30 repetitions
See pg. 168, photo 60, a-c

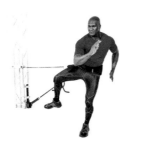

8. **Standing hip abduction with elastic resistance**
20 repetitions
See pg. 172, photo 62, a-d

PLEASE NOTE:

1. Weights, band thickness, and repetitions must be customized for each individual client.

2. 2-33 lbs. = low | 33-44 lbs. = medium | 44-55 lbs. = high

3. Level 1 = 3 sets | Level 2 = 5 sets | Level 3 = 7 sets

LAMAR SYSTEM WORKOUT 2

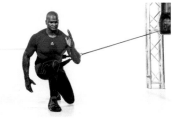

1. Wheel lunge against resistance
20 repetitions
See pg. 184, photo 68, a-d

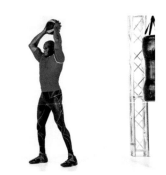

2. Overhead chop with medicine ball
30 repetitions
See pg. 162, photo 57, a-d

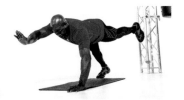

3. Plank – alternating arm and leg extensions
20 repetitions
See pg. 154, photo 53, a-b

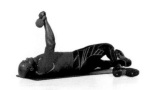

4. Kettlebell floor press – extended range
25 repetitions
See pg. 142, photo 47, a-b

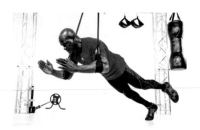

5. Plank – leg lifts with sling trainer
20 repetitions
See pg. 166, photo 59, a-b

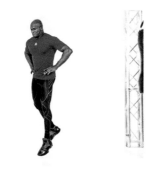

6. Split lunge jumps
20 repetitions
See pg. 192, photo 72, a-d

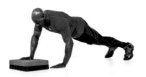

7. Hand step-ups on unstable surfaces
25 repetitions
See pg. 148, photo 50, a-e

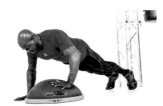

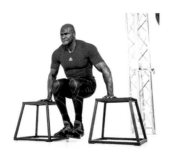

8. Squat hold
1 minute
See pg. 146, photo 49, a-b

PLEASE NOTE:
1. Weights, band thickness, and repetitions must be customized for each individual client.
2. 2-33 lbs. = low | 33-44 lbs. = medium | 44-55 lbs. = high
3. Level 1 = 3 sets | Level 2 = 5 sets | Level 3 = 7 sets

LAMAR SYSTEM WORKOUT 3

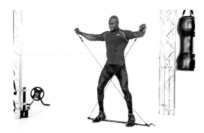

1. Lateral raise with resistance
25 repetitions
See pg. 140, photo 46, a-c

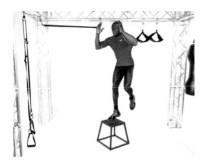

2. Upward jump
20 repetitions
See pg. 170, photo 61, a-c

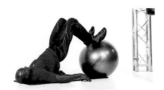

3. Leg curls with large fitness ball
30 repetitions
See pg. 182, photo 67, a-d

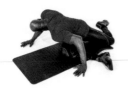

4. Supine hip adduction with elastic resistance
25 repetitions
See pg. 188, photo 70, a-c

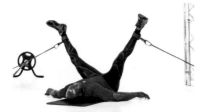

5. Side twist hip stretch
20 repetitions
See pg. 176, photo 64, a-d

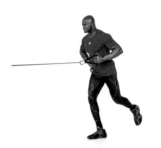

6. Standing pull (single leg)
20 repetitions
See pg. 203, photo 77, f-g

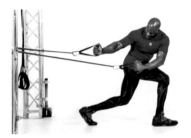

7. Standing pull (lunge)
20 repetitions
See pg. 204, photo 78, e-g

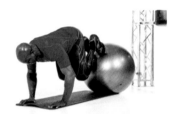

8. Downward-facing knee bends
30 repetitions
See pg. 215, photo 93, a-b

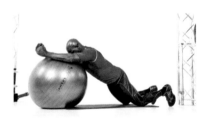

9. Roll out
15 repetitions
See pg. 209, photo 84, a-b

PLEASE NOTE:

1. The stability ball allows you to specifically target different back muscles—the small muscles that stabilize as well as the large ones that primarily facilitate movements.
2. Level 1 = 3 sets | Level 2 = 5 sets | Level 3 = 7 sets

LAMAR SYSTEM WORKOUT 4

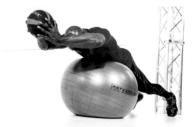

1. Hyperextension with medicine ball
20 repetitions
See pg. 104, photo 28, a-b

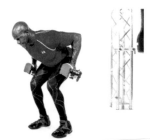

2. Hyperextension, leg extension with large fitness ball
25 repetitions
See pg. 100, photo 26, a-c

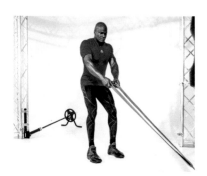

3. Shrugs with elastic band
30 repetitions
See pg. 110, photo 31, a-e

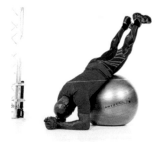

4. Two-arm row with dumbbells
20 repetitions
See pg. 120, photo 36, a-c

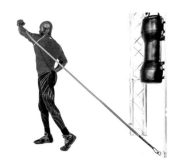

5. Twisted press with elastic band resistance
20 repetitions
See pg. 136, photo 44, a-b

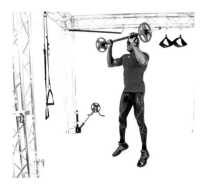

6. Jerk, split
20 repetitions
See pg. 138, photo 45, a-d

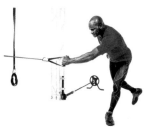

7. Standing pull
20 repetitions
See pg. 204, photo 78, c-d

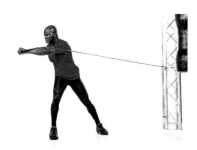

8. Press in standing position
20 repetitions
See pg. 207, photo 81, a-b

PLEASE NOTE:
Level 1 = 3 sets | Level 2 = 5 sets | Level 3 = 7 sets

LAMAR SYSTEM FITNESS BALL WORKOUT

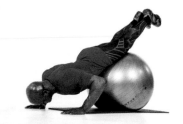

1. Push-up
25 repetitions
See pg. 207, photo 82, a-b

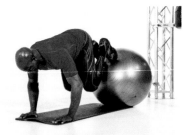

2. Downward-facing knee bends
25 repetitions
See pg. 215, photo 93, a-b

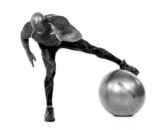

3. Side squat
25 repetitions
See pg. 212, photo 88, a-b

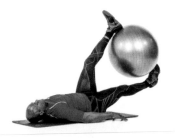

4. Leg scissors
20 repetitions
See pg. 214, photo 92, a-b

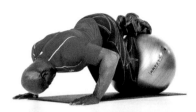

5. Push-up variations
20 repetitions
See pg. 208, photo 83, a-b

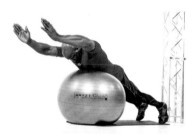

6. Roll out
20 repetitions
See pg. 209, photo 84, a-b

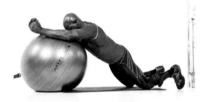

7. Trunk extension
20 repetitions
See pg. 213, photo 89, a-b

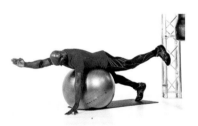

8. Contralateral superman
3 x 1 minute per side
See pg. 213, photo 90, a-b

PLEASE NOTE:
Level 1 = 3 sets | Level 2 = 5 sets | Level 3 = 7 sets

LAMAR SYSTEM STROOPS, STIK, AND SLING TRAINER WORKOUTS

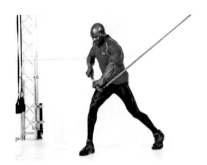

1. Lift/chop
25 repetitions
See pg. 217-218, photo 69, a-c

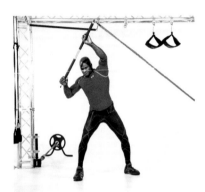

2. Circles/rotations
20 repetitions
See pg. 219, photo 97, a-c

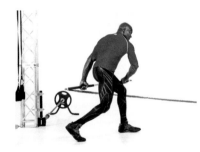

3. Row
20 repetitions
See pg. 220-221, photo 98, a-c

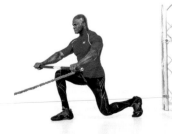

4. Lunge variation
20 repetitions
See pg. 222, photos 99 a-c

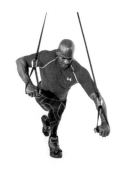

5. Arm push
15 repetitions
See pg. 223, photo 100, a-c

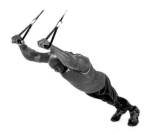

6. Reverse pull-up
15 repetitions

See pg. 224, photo 102, a-c

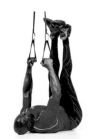

7. Extension
20 repetitions
See pg. 224, photo 101, a-b

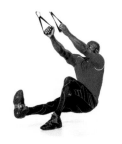

8. Pistol squat/knee bend
20 repetitions
See pg. 225, photo 103, a-b

PLEASE NOTE:
1. Band thickness and repetitions must be customized for each individual client.
2. Level 1 = 3 sets | Level 2 = 5 sets | Level 3 = 7 sets

LAMAR SYSTEM CORE TRAINER WORKOUT

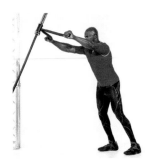

1. Shoulder press
20 repetitions
See pg. 227-228, photo 105, a-d

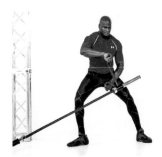

2. Twisted push, standing
15 repetitions
See pg. 228-229, photo 106, a-d

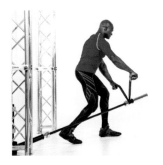

3. Reverse push
15 repetitions
See pg. 229-230, photos 107 a-e

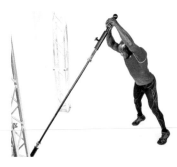

4. Squat – push – rotation
20 repetitions
See pg. 233, photo 110, a-d

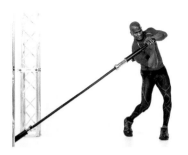

5. Upper cuts
20 repetitions
See pg. 234, photo 111, a-c

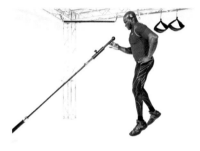

6. Single-arm clean and jerk
20 repetitions
See pg. 235, photo 112, a-d

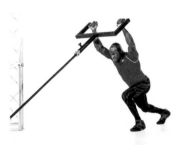

7. Push
20 repetitions
See pg. 239, photo 115, a-c

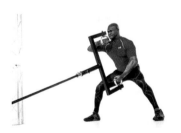

8. Lateral steps
20 repetitions
See pg. 240, photo 116, a-c

PLEASE NOTE:

1. Intensify these exercises by adding additional plates to the bar.
2. Weights start at 3 pounds. Added weight depends on client.
3. Level 1 = 3 sets | Level 2 = 5 sets | Level 3 = 7 sets

REFERENCES

American College of Sports Medicine: *ACSM's Advanced Exercise Physiology* (2006). Philadelphia: Lippincott Williams&Wilki.

Baechle, T. R. & Earle, W. R. (2003): *Essentials of Personal Training.* Champaign: Human Kinetics.

Baechle, T. R. & Earle, W. R. (2000): *Essentials of Strength Training and Conditioning* (2nd Edition). Champaign: Human Kinetics.

Bear, M., Connors, B. & Paradiso, M. (2006): *Neurosience. Explore the Brain.* (3rd Edition). Lippincott Williams and Wilkins: Baltimore.

Brown, L. E. & Ferrigno, V. (Hrsg.) (2005): *Training for Speed, Agility and Quickness: Training Drills for Peak Performance.* Champaign: Human Kinetics.

Bruhn, S. & Gollhofer, A. (2001). Neurophysiologische Grundlagen der Propriozeption und Sensomotorik. *Med.Orth.Techn.*, 121, 66-71.

Crossley, J. (2013): *Personal Training: Theory and Practice* (2nd Edition). Abingdon: Routledge.

Goleman, D. (1995): *Emotional Intelligence. Why it can matter more than IQ.* New York: Bantam Books.

Jemmett , R. (2003): *Spinal stabilization – The new science of back pain* (2nd Edition). Minneapolis: Orthopedic Physical Therapy Products.

Kent, G. & Carr, R.: Comparative Anatomy of the Vertebrates. 9th Edition. New York: McGraw-Hill Science/Engineering/Math.

Marras, W. & Karwowski, W. (2006): Fundamentals and Assessment Tools for Occupational Ergonomics. Boca Raton: CRC Press.

Penedo, F. J. & Dahn, J. R. (2005): Exercise and well-being: a review of mental and physical health benefits associated with physical activity. *Curr Opin Psychiatry.* 18(2): 189-93.

Poirier P., Despres J. P. (2001): Exercise in weight management of obesity. *Cardiol Clin.* 19(3): 459-70.

Riemann, B. L. & Lephart, S. M. (2002): The Sensorimotor System, Part I: The Physiologic Basis of Functional Joint Stability. *J Athl Train* 37(1). 71-79.

Voight, M. L. (2007): *Musculoskeletal Interventions: Techniques for Therapeutic Exercise.* Mcgraw-Hill Professional.

Warburton D.E., Nicol, C. W. & Bredin S. S. (2006): Health benefits of physical activity: the evidence. *CMAJ.* 14. 174(6): 801-9.

Winter, D. A.: Human balance and posture control during standing and walking (1995). *Gait & Posture* (3). 193-214.

FURTHER READING

http://physics.info/

http://www.emedicinehealth.com/anatomy_of_the_central_nervous_system/article_em.htm

http://accessphysiotherapy.mhmedical.com/content.aspx?bookid=960&sectionid=53549687

https://en.wikipedia.org/wiki/David_H._Hubel

http://www.bodyworlds.com/Downloads/did_you_know.pdf

http://www.britannica.com/science/human-skeletal-system

http://www.mnsu.edu/emuseum/biology/humananatomy/skeletal/skeletalsystem.html

http://csep10.phys.utk.edu/astr161/lect/history/newton3laws.html

http://hyperphysics.phy-astr.gsu.edu/hbase/newt.html

ACKNOWLEDGMENTS

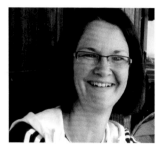

Many thanks to Astrid Buscher for her exceptional effort and outstanding support during our collaboration on the Lamar Lowery's Functional Fitness project.

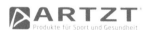

A big thank you to the Ludwig Artzt GmbH for a fantastic collaboration and for providing the functional small equipment for the Lamar Lowery Functional Fitness project. I look forward to working with you again in the future.

Many thanks to the entire Meyer & Meyer publishing house for the excellent cooperation! What a great team!

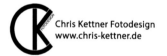

I've enjoyed working with Chris Kettner Fotodesign, who is always professional, reliable, competent, and honest. And he has a keen eye for the perfect shot.

Thank you, Chris!

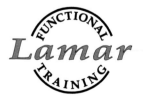

I have now completed my first book project. It is my hope that everyone can take something away from this to live a healthier life. Enjoy Functional Fitness – The Personal Trainer's Guide!

CREDITS

Illustrations
Pg. 48, 50, 56 Sarah Ewald

Editing
Elizabeth Evans

Photos
Chris Kettner Fotosdesign
Philipp Artzt

Pg. 68 h/p cosmos

Pg. 8, 14, 42, 53, 79, 90 © Thinkstock

Layout and cover design
Eva Feldmann

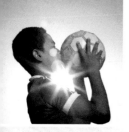
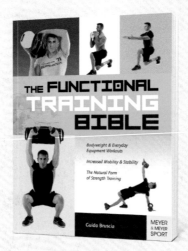

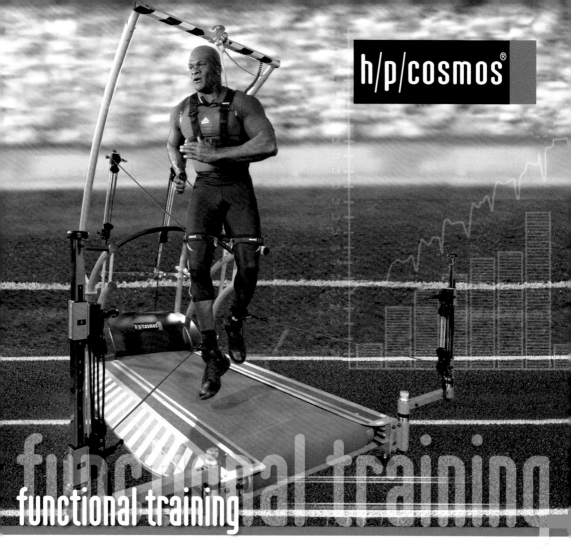

h/p/cosmos®

functional training

with high performance treadmill pulsar® 3p & robowalk®

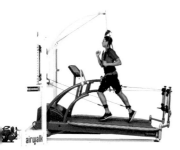

h/p/cosmos treadmill pulsar® 3p with robowalk® expander and unweighting system airwalk® ap

Videos:

The h/p/cosmos high performance treadmill pulsar® 3p in combination with the robowalk® expander is perfect for functional training on the treadmill:

▌ dynamic workout of the upper and lower body!

▌ interval-training and hill-sprints with reproducable settings

▌ large running surface of 190 x 65 cm (74.8 x 25.59")

▌ speeds of up to 40 km/h (standard, optional 45 km/h ~ 28 mph)

▌ over-frequency training with the airwalk® ap unweighting system

▌ training and activation of the anterior, posterior and lateral chain with robowalk® / roborun®

▌ core-stabilization training while running on the treadmill

☎ +49 86 69 86 42 0   sales@h-p-cosmos.com   www.h-p-cosmos.com   ahead of time®